BODY AND MIND IN HARMONY

T'ai Chi Ch'üan

(Wu Style)

An Ancient Chinese Way of Exercise

BY

SOPHIA DELZA

DRAWINGS BY THE AUTHOR

Library of Congress Catalogue Card Number: 60-14596

First edition

Manufactured in the United States of America

●

The quotations throughout the text are mainly from the *T'ai Chi Ch'üan Ching* (Classic) attributed to Wang Chung-Yueh of the Ming Dynasty.

To C. A. G.
who made it possible for me to live in China

ACKNOWLEDGMENTS

The author will always feel grateful to her teacher in China, Mr. Ma Yüeh-Liang, the great master of T‘ai Chi Ch‘üan, for having imparted his knowledge to her with such generosity.

She would like particularly to thank Mr. Koo Hsien-Liang, whose scholarly and sensitively artistic translations of Chinese classics helped her immeasurably and who so sympathetically supported her activities.

She is also grateful to Mr. Chang Kuo-Ho, of the United Nations, who suggested that she do the book on T‘ai Chi Ch‘üan; the San Francisco T‘ai Chi Ch‘üan Club for their warm sponsorship of her performances; Joseph Carter, of the *New York Times;* Nina Gordani for her personal management of the author's performance-lectures; and Hubert Wang, who translated Chinese literature for her.

And especially, the author is happy to acknowledge the honor the members of the United Nations' T‘ai Chi Ch‘üan Club have done her by asking her to teach them. There are too many to mention all, but those of the original group are: Hsü Ming-Chen, Djang Chu, Edward Lai, Shih Tao-Tsi, Tsao Hung-Chao, Shen Chang-Jui, Yen Cheng, Wellington Lee (present president), Robert Mok, Booker Lee, and Simon Chang.

CONTENTS

PART I

THE
T'AI
CHI
CH'ÜAN
WAY

INTRODUCTION

"What is past one cannot amend,
For the future one can always provide."
—From the *Analects* of Confucius

Is there anyone in the world whose idea of being truly healthy would not include, along with a healthy body, a fine mind combined with an ease of disposition? Fleeting glimpses of this feeling of harmony are experienced by everyone at some time in his life. In our colloquialisms we see revealed the inner clear relationship of mind and body. "I feel as if I were floating" is a common expression to describe a peak of contentment of physical comfort. Well-being produces a sensation of lightness where the body is sensed but not felt. "I'm simply walking on air" is an image that almost obliterates the body and makes the spirit seem all powerful.

What an agony of indecision and what physical immobility are exposed in "I'm all tied up in knots." "My heart stood still" expresses an anxiety that almost strangles the circulation. Composure and mental equilibrium can hardly be sustained in a weak and unhealthy system where discomfort dominates the consciousness.

The effect of body on mind and mind on body is in evidence at every turn of our lives every day. The realization of this fact is a step toward making an effort to find a technique that can "nourish the body and calm the spirit"—a technique that, as an exercise, can give action to thought, and, as a philosophy, can give thought to action, and which as a composite art is so synthesized as to make the whole greater than the sum of its intriguing parts.

Such is T'ai Chi Ch'üan (pronounced Tye Gee Chwan), the

unique Chinese System of Soft-Intrinsic Exercise, which, dating back to A.D. 1000, is extremely popular today. In the present century four T'ai Chi Ch'üan styles (P'ai) are being practiced: Yang, Wu, Ho, Sun. Illustrated in this book is *Wu*, a style that concentrates on harmonious self-development with the philosophical as well as the psychological aspects emphasized. It has as its goal the achievement of health and tranquillity by means of a "way of movement," characterized by a technique of moving slowly and continuously, without strain, through a varied sequence of contrasting forms that create stable vitality with calmness, balanced strength with flexibility, controlled energy with awareness.

There is a significant difference in concept between the dance-art that is used as an exercise and the exercise that is an art in itself. As a modern dancer I appreciate this, having created dance forms for the purpose of art and for exercise. Designed movements, patterns, and excerpts of dance techniques, which are extracted from the dance-art for use as general exercise, though inevitably stimulating and enlivening, must be considered inadequate for the more profound, permanent aspect of the development of mind and body.

T'ai Chi Ch'üan is not a by-product, as it were, of any other art-dance form; it is not derived from ancient Chinese commemorative dance, folk, or classical Chinese theater dance, and does not resemble them in dynamics, rhythm, or structure. T'ai Chi Ch'üan is a complete entity, composed to answer the needs to which it is directed. Total in concept, it is a synthesis of form and function. With the elements of structure and movement so consummately composed, it is an art in the deepest sense of the word. Aesthetically, it can be compared to a composition by Bach or a Shakespearean sonnet. However, T'ai Chi Ch'üan is not art directed outward to an audience. It is an art-in-action for the doer; the observer, moved by its beauty, can only surmise its content. The *experience* of the form in process of change makes it an art for the self.

My intention in writing this book is to bring to the attention of Western people this ancient masterpiece of health exercise, which, ancient though it is, is supremely suitable for us all in these modern times. I wish to create an informed understanding of what is necessary, theoretically, for a vital life, and also to arouse the interest of the reader and his willingness to apply this exercise for his own use. As an exercise that demands no physical strength to begin with, it therefore is as good for the weak as for the well, for young and old, men and women. Since the techniques are adjusted to, and develop with, individual capacities, it is practical for any disposition.

Movement by movement, step by step, with its organic and intrinsic harmony, it trains both body and mind—to longer life with heightened interest and deeper understanding. The calmness that comes from harmonious physical activity and mental perception, and the composure that comes from deep feeling and comprehension are the very heart of this exercise.

The wonderful thing about writing a book on this subject is that its always-to-be applied principles are constantly with one, under one's very fingers, for immediate use. When one is blooming and content, to practice it gives greater growth and awareness. When, working restlessly, impatiently, one has come to an impasse, then to do the exercise is revivifying; it settles the mind, quiets the spirit, smoothes out the emotions; and with refreshened mind and unagitated heart, one can take on problems again (as has been the experience of many students in diverse fields of work).

The deep interest and enthusiasm that T'ai Chi Ch'üan has aroused in those who practice it and those who have seen it have also contributed to my desire to make it available for those who have no teacher. It is a preparation for those who will study with someone eventually, because it is best "that beginners be guided by oral teaching, but nevertheless, if you direct yourself with diligence, skill will take care of itself" (as stated in *T'ai Chi Ch'üan Ching,* Classic of the Ming Dynasty). For those who are studying or have studied, it can be a permanent record for more profound self-study. ". . . in teaching others everything depends on consistency, for it is only through repetition that the pupil makes the material his own" (*I-Ching,* Book of Changes).

Needless to say, there are a great many books on T'ai Chi Ch'üan by Chinese writers that deal with its philosophical, practical, historical, and physiological aspects in a most thorough and masterful way. Then you may well ask what is my contribution, if it is a contribution.

In the light of what Chinese literature contains, this book must indeed be considered modest. Let me mention at this point that I have omitted certain features not imperative for the Western student as a beginner. Those are the techniques and skills that the study of this exercise can lead to, such as the Art of Self-Defense and Joint Hand Operations.

I do not touch upon a very important subject, that of *Ch'i,* variously interpreted as breath, spirit, or air and as the nervous system in the latest books. The doctrine of the use of Ch'i is an important element that enters into the philosophy of art, aesthetics, science, and philosophy. Ch'i is a *vital* force differentiated from *life* force; it is the rhythm of nature, the creative principle that makes life. It is circulation and the circular movement of breath within one, an aspect that T'ai Chi Ch'üan is greatly concerned with, at an advanced stage of development. Ch'i, as "an urge or energy, compounded of spirit and in a mysterious way the physical breath" (E. Herbert in *Taoist Notebook*), I leave as a subject to be studied with the masters of T'ai Chi Ch'üan.

In rendering the entire exercise precisely, I have included innumerable details that are not noted in Chinese versions, because there they are taken for granted for reasons that are obvious. We, in the West, with no background for these techniques, cultural or actual, require more specific, minute, exacting explanations with a more *simplified* analysis. I have, so to speak, put the microscope on the action, without reinterpreting or changing it. Certain repetitions are unavoidable and perhaps are necessary, to open up new perspectives and perceptions.

The Chinese people are prepared philosophically and psychologically for the theory and practice of T'ai Chi Ch'üan. An accepted method of movement, it is available everywhere; they have only to reach out for it, to walk to the park (literally), and it can be learned. The degree to which we in the West are *not* prepared for it has governed the choice of the material in this book. In doing so I have kept in mind that an old Chinese idea of proven values is being presented in a new western environment.

The principles, qualities, and features inherent in the nature of this exercise are faithfully given, as taught to me by my teacher Mr. Ma Yüeh-Liang. However, I have expatiated upon them in order to clarify and emphasize their content. I have consciously included personal aesthetic and psychological interpretations, which have inevitably come from my increasing experience with this exercise, and which are the result of my inquiring into related fields of study and of discussion with T'ai Chi Ch'üan experts.

WHAT T'AI CHI CH'ÜAN IS

T'ai Chi Ch'üan is a form of Ch'üan. To call T'ai Chi Ch'üan Body and Mind in Harmony is to state its essence in a few succinct words. In *T'ai Chi Ch'üan—An Ancient Chinese Way of Exercise to Achieve Health and Tranquillity,* its nature is indicated in terms of the objectives to be reached. But only by translating T'ai Chi Ch'üan literally do we give it its real significance; in so doing it becomes more than a definition—it becomes this book.

What is Ch'üan? Ch'üan means fist, metaphorically action, a word that connotes power and control over one's own actions: the epitome of organized movement and the ultimate in protection of the self. To be expert in Ch'üan is to have immunity—immunity from destructive external forces and from poor health. It is also to have the power to control the self. The uses of this power and the ends toward which it is to be directed depend entirely upon the inclinations and interests of the individual; these may range from the purely physical to the philosophic or spiritual.

To us in the West, a fist provocatively denotes aggressive attack. A fisted hand, on the contrary, in terms of ancient Chinese thought, meant concentration, isolation, and containment, as depicted in wood blocks showing figures in various exercising positions (Kung-Fu) with fisted hands. We can assume that Ch'üan implies the active as controlled by the inactive—the active being form or matter and the inactive being spirit or mind.

As a synonym for exercise, with deep implications as to its usefulness, Ch'üan is a technique of organized harmonious forms. Its essence is continuity of action where each movement evolves from and grows out of what it is joined to, which spurs on and motivates the oncoming movement. The correspondence between the parts of the body is essential to structure, idea, and feeling. "One single movement suffices to affect other movements." "No isolated rest without eventually enveloping the whole." "Just as in the turning flow of a stream, so the positions are determined by the spaces between."

Symbolically, Ch'üan is mental and physical co-ordination. If the body is in fine health, then the mind can function skillfully and adroitly. The body is the form, and the mind, which is the spirit, is actually the moving force. Mental "motion" is present with every physical action. T'ai Chi Ch'üan is "controlled by the mind" exercise (*Ting Tou Yuan*).

What is T'ai Chi? T'ai Chi is the concept that all of life is comprised of, and has been set in motion by, the constant interplay of two vital energies, Yin the passive, and Yang the active principle. "T'ai Chi is the mother of Yin and Yang [everything female and male]," which has given rise to everything under the sun.

No part has a life of its own, but each exists in complementary interaction with the other. "Yin and Yang mutually help each other." "T'ai Chi is the root of motion (Yang) which has division, and of stillness (Yin) which has union." T'ai Chi *is* this duality in harmonious relationship.

The symbol for the T'ai Chi is a circle divided into two curved shapes of equal size, one being Yin, the shadowed right part, the other Yang, the light part. A touch of Yin in Yang and of Yang in Yin is indicated by the small spot or dot of the opposite color in each area, showing the flexible and sympathetic character of each to the other. The line between them has the movement of a wave. The fall and rise of the wave-line is also Yin and Yang, and this flowing is restrained and contained by the evenness of the circumference. All of this movement represents the continuity of the life force, which is *movement.*

Yin as the receptive, feminine, and Yang as the creative, masculine, complement each other. Though opposite, they are not in opposition or antagonistic. Though different, they supplement each other. In the continuous movement between them, without beginning and without end, when Yang reaches its final moment, then Yin is created and starts when Yang is completed. The interplay of these two fundamental and vital elements implies "perpetual motion." Together, in T'ai Chi where their relationship is perfect; they constitute equilibrium and harmony.

T'ai Chi holds in balance what is separated. A few examples of the opposites (placing the Yang before the Yin) as experienced in the exercise of T'ai Chi Ch'üan, are: movement-stillness, motion-rest, tangible-intangible, straight-curved, expansion-contraction, inhalation-exhalation, outside-inside, solid-empty (void), light-dark, firm-soft, open-closed, right-left, forward-backward, float-settle, and rise-sink. There is nothing without its opposite; there is nothing that does not change (move) in order to be permanent (to live)—which in itself is a Yin-Yang statement.

We in the West are apt to overexert ourselves in exercise and sports, believing that a hard and tense movement indicates strength and control, and that power comes from the ability to expend energy violently. The spirit of T'ai Chi Ch'üan is the antithesis of such a point of view. With the technique of T'ai Chi Ch'üan, true energy can be controlled, strength balanced, and vitality increased, by using the body in such a way so as *not* to strain the muscles, *not* to overactivate the heart, *not* to exert oneself excessively. It is in the philosophy of T'ai Chi Ch'üan that in order to prolong the life of the body, to stabilize the life of the emotions, and to intensify the life of the mind, conscious co-operation of the mind with activity is a deep necessity. For certainly peace of mind cannot be attained without the use of the mind. The consideration of man's total health as an inseparable unity is evident in every moment of this long, slow exercise.

BENEFITS

The practice of T'ai Chi Ch'üan is a way to develop both body and mind to such a degree that "one can retard old age and make spring eternal." At the same time as it strengthens and revitalizes the body, it helps "the cultivation of a calm heart," and enables the mind to function with more awareness, clarity, and concentration.

T'ai Chi Ch'üan as a physical exercise increases the blood circulation and activity of the glands, nourishes muscles, facilitates joint-action, stimulates the nervous system, all without increasing the activity of the heart or breathing rhythm. The technique, circular in nature, soft, slow, and continuous, and above all subscribing to the principles of Yin and Yang, affects the entire system in a superior way, involving every organ as well as the surface skin. T'ai Chi Ch'üan properly harmonizes the circulation of the various vital currents and, so to speak, unties the knots or pressures blocking the process of assimilation.

As a healing art, T'ai Chi Ch'üan serves as a remedy for high blood pressure, anemia, joint diseases, and gastic disturbances, and has been used as a cure for tuberculosis.

T'ai Chi Ch'üan aims also at "the cultivation of temperament." The balance of movements and the way of using slowness, lightness, and calmness relax nervous temperaments, give one an easy pace and "therefore a good disposition," and "rid one of arrogance and conceit." Because every movement is anticipated by the mind, patience and control of temper develop without effort, and a consistent equilibrium between the heart and mind is established.

We know very well that dynamic interest is beneficial to one's nervous system, and that a happy spirit and an enthusiastic frame of mind can affect health favorably. And being in a state of good health can exhilarate one's spirits. With a good nervous system one's whole being becomes more perceptive, alert, and receptive.

The benefits of T'ai Chi Ch'üan are intellectual and psychological, too. One can more easily adjust oneself to meet the various and continuously changing stimuli of one's environment with steady equanimity.

With an increase of intrinsic energy, one's interest is heightened. Because the techniques involve change and nuance, awareness and mental alertness, one becomes more sensitive and capable of greater understanding. The mind is concentrated. This basic principle of concentration where the mind directs the energy and the energy in turn exercises the body, is a key factor in attaining the final objectives: acquiring energy without tenseness, strength without hardness, vitality without nervousness, and especially achieving tranquillity. This is not the tranquillity of inaction, but the tranquillity of the following definition from *I-Ching*, Book of Changes:

> Tranquillity is a kind of vigilant attention. It is when tranquillity is perfect that the human faculties display all their resources, because [then] they are enlightened by reason and sustained by knowledge.

This definition sums up the Chinese point of view, essential in the study of T'ai Chi Ch'üan.

CHARACTERISTICS OF THE WAY OF MOVEMENT

The technique of T'ai Chi Ch'üan is based on a way of movement that significantly involves the Forms, with a styled method of making the pattern evolve from the movement, and the movement from the Forms.

The structures are so varied as to put into play every part of the body from the smallest joint to the largest muscle. Harmoniously designed, masterfully patterned, they are done with flowing continuity. Slowness, evenness, clarity, balance, and calmness are the five basic qualities of its composite technique. The perfect weaving of the dynamics of movement and form promotes fine circulation, and, above all, quiets the mind and regulates the emotions.

In the first place, it is the "softness" of this style of exercise (see page 14) which develops energy, by never allowing one to expend oneself in a gesture of finality. This softness contrasts with the hard or overenergetic force that does *not* permit such reserve of action. Natural body behavior with a style of moving in fluid and continuous motion "like the movement of a never-ending river" eliminates any possibility of becoming rigid or hard.

The great play of dynamics as contained in T'ai Chi is so utilized in this exercise that no one part of the body can be overstrained. Because of this constant alternating interplay of action, one's whole system feels neither a beginning nor an end of movement, from which a state of emotional equilibrium is created.

The immense variety of patterns keeps one mentally stimulated as the techniques develop from Form to Form. The mind cannot be anywhere *but* on the action since the variations and repetitions demand total attention. Because the structure does not evolve correctly without this mind participation, control of the consciousness develops inevitably. Concentration is a natural result of such technique and form.

Moving in slow time prevents the body from becoming tense or hard and makes muscles resilient and pliable. Strength cannot be wasted or falsely propelled, because slow movement requires attentive control.

The entire system is warmed up gradually as the action accumulates. Patterns and movements, in subtle succession, activate different parts of the body, and never at any time repeat themselves in overconcentrated units. This enables the body to do more without making the heart beat faster to keep up with the body changes.

Breathing is natural—light or deep depending on the structure and the positions of the Forms themselves. However, beginners must not concern themselves with the breathing process. This aspect is developed in the advanced study of T'ai Chi Ch'üan.

The fundamentally slow and unvarying basic tempo contributes to the ability to sustain conscious control and aids in building up reserves of energy. With the flowing alternation of light and strong dynamic, of void and solid forms, circulation is made to move freely to all parts of the body.

The movement requires that motion be outwardly unvarying and in continuous flow. Ability to maintain a consistently slow tempo and an even quality over a long period of time is an indication, not only that the body has acquired strength and control, but also that the mind is in harmony with the action.

Personal moods and distracting emotions evaporate as you are taken out of yourself by your attention to motion and forms that are completely objective and impersonal. In this way, you are taken into yourself, into understanding yourself without subjective interference.

In terms of pure movement, the patterns are so constructed that the strong alternates with the light, the active with the quiescent, the weighted with the empty, the solid with the void, expansion with contraction—the relationships being as flexible and continuous as the form of the wave line within the T'ai Chi.

Within a design, one part of the body may be still while another part is active; one hand in a Yin position and the other Yang. All the weight, with controlled force, may be held on one side, while the other is light and receptive, an opposite relationship taking place in the following sequence, with differently designed arrangements. No muscle, joint, limb, no part of the body is ever overtaxed or underactivated. Both excess and deficiency are avoided, since each is contrary to the philosophy of T'ai Chi Ch'üan.

STRUCTURE (YIN-YANG)

Not only are the elements of Yin-Yang apparent in the movement and design from pattern to pattern, no matter how minute, but they are contained also in the structure of the Forms, which are composites of many designs.

In going from one design to another the connecting line is so deliberately controlled that it is as smooth, as unvarying, as continuous as a circle. Though the Form is constantly changing from Yin to Yang, the external appearance never shows that there are changes in the dynamics of muscular tension. In this "soft-intrinsic" exercise, the outer appearance is soft, and the inner force is firm, whereas in "hard-extrinsic" exercise, the dynamics, always intense, are never varied.

Yin-Yang appears in the exerciser's attitude as well. The strength used to manipulate the body is not registered on the face; the spirit is calm, and, therefore, the face is quiet and the look is effortless. This is *not* deception. It is exactly how one feels, because the intrinsic nature of this technique gives the doer the feeling of containment while he is being active.

Because the inner control that the action demands is not apparent to the observer, the action seems weightless, airy, easy, thoughtless, and soft without energy. But the weightlessness actually is of such substance that "motion is like refined steel." What seems to be easy is "as controlled as a hawk trying to catch a rabbit." It is "as thoughtless as a cat waiting to catch a mouse" where attention and concentration are completely centered. The softness has "the reserve of energy of a bow about to be snapped." Inside one is firm, stable, controlled, and at the same time the appearance is of repose and effortlessness. This is Yin-Yang in its relation to the outside world.

HARMONY OF BODY AND MIND

The way of movement is, in a deeper sense, related to the "movement of the mind"; the mind must direct the body movement; the mind wills and the body behaves. The alertness and concentration needed to do this are developed as the Forms are being mastered.

One of the great advantages of T'ai Chi Ch'üan is that one can never be automatic when doing it. The body and personality are one in action. The benefit of this is perhaps obvious, since T'ai Chi Ch'üan has, as one of its goals, the development of awareness and consciousness, quickened reflexes, and an alert mind.

The mind can be directed to control the body at a fraction of a moment's notice. The action is so designed that the logical follow-through is upset if the mind absents itself. The astutely composed themes and the artful arrangements of detailed designs bring the attention back from its undirected wanderings, forcing one to be doubly attentive. This is truly an exercise *with* the mind, training it to function consistently and harmoniously with the will.

To omit any of the repeated Forms, in addition to weakening the mental concept of T'ai Chi Ch'üan, will ruin its structure, which has philosophical and artistic meaning. The composition of the structure is explicit as to floor pattern, space, and form.

The structure arouses a sense of aesthetic appreciation, a satisfaction that comes from the balanced harmony of a perfectly arranged work of art. The repeated forms, spaced with psychological insight, give mental rest and physical ease, because at certain points in the development of the exercise, it is necessary *not* to have a new problem. The exercise ends exactly in the footprints where it started. The significance of T'ai Chi Ch'üan's ending and starting as it does is that it gives to the performer a sense of the whole, which, though completed, inevitably resumes its motion.

The co-ordination aspect of movement within movement and design within design demands complete attention. The subtle regulation of the timing of each small part within the whole *is* co-ordination. The mind moves from form, to style, to tempo, to co-ordination, to plasticity, to dynamics, to "feeling," and yet seems to acknowledge all at the same time. Concentrated by this variety, mind, attention, and awareness are one.

The mental habit of concentration acquired from these techniques is easily carried over to other subjects, which is another way of saying that when mind and body are in harmony, anything that must be done, can be done with the complete co-operation of mind, will, and feeling. The techniques of T'ai Chi Ch'üan give thought to action and action to thought with the mind in control. The profound and minutely brilliant detail in the exercise patterns will prod you, coax you, and lead you into the clear path of heightened awareness. Awareness overcomes restlessness. The act of consciously focusing attention can, almost instantly, make you calm, when in action or at rest.

TWO INTRINSIC PRINCIPLES: SOFTNESS AND CIRCULAR MOVEMENT

Softness

This "inner" or soft school of movement can easily be recognized by the fact that there is no visible exertion in the execution of the movements. The action and the person appear to be completely relaxed, because the activity is hidden inside, below the surface. The continuous flow of movement into movement, without straining, also contributes to this outer "soft" appearance. Actually all the movements are done with controlled inner force. It is not the extent to which movement can go that matters; rather it is the quality in reserve that determines its softness, which means "intrinsic-stored-up-within." With this soft technique the body can be held loosely and circulation is, therefore, unrestricted. This helps store up intrinsic energy and makes an elasticity which is "inside and yet is rich in power of resilience."

With continuity and slowness as component parts of softness, calmness and lightness are the inevitable results. No matter what the movements—pushing, pressing, lifting, stretching, leg-lifts, or deep charges—because of this development of soft elasticity, the breath never comes quickly, nor is the heart beat accelerated. Flexibility and vigor are developed without forced effort.

Circular Movement

T'ai Chi Ch'üan is often referred to as the circular exercise because all patterns and designs (with the obvious necessary exceptions) are composed of circles, curves, arcs, parabolas, and spirals of all sizes, which go in many directions—horizontal, vertical, or slanted. They may move in opposition or concurrently, and in various tempi.

This technique is not arbitrary or just abstractly decorative. The act of weaving and interrelating the patterns in a circular way evokes calmness and creates energy. By limiting the extent of the action, circular motion helps to reserve energy. It prevents one from overexpending oneself, since the dynamics of physical tension can be controlled when moving in a line of a curve. The sustained ability to move continuously in a curve increases strength and endurance.

Circular motion, where there appears to be no ending to the gestures and no corners to the designs, creates evenness, which is an important factor in relaxing the tenseness of body and mind. A circle of movement produces a sense of detachment, containment, and emotional security.

All the diverse circular units in the exercise are balanced by evenly paced action and by the control of the center of gravity. This combination resembles the symbol for T'ai Chi, in which the outer circle equilibrates the movement within it. By maintaining the circular smoothness in action, an outer passivity is attained. Simultaneously, to "balance the opposites," with the activity of the movements, an inner stillness is created.

From doing T'ai Chi Ch'üan one gets the feeling of perpetual motion. The circle and all its varying forms hold the movements together in a unity of technique and mood. The basic tempo remains unchanged and holds together other varying tempi, which are slower, thus integrating form and space. The space in which the body moves, precisely designed, is regulated by the patterns of the body composition. Although there is continuing motion, the action is so distributed that no *single* part of the body is in continual motion, or is continually at rest. The Yin-Yang elements, alternating with regularity, give an impetus to the motion. Here, too, the dynamics of lightness and force, moving from one part of the body to another, keep the action continuous and perpetual.

The body in action is a small universe of multiple movements and synchronized Forms, moving on itself and in space, duplicating, as it were, the composite rotation of the planets, where each, turning in its own rhythm, is in perfect co-ordination with the others in orbit.

FIVE ESSENTIAL QUALITIES

Slowness, lightness, clarity, balance, and calmness are each the cause and effect of the other. The inner essence and the outer style, the means and the end, are harmoniously one. Through their fluent interplay, the form and spirit of T'ai Chi Ch'üan is crystallized.

Slowness (Man)

It is absolutely essential to move slowly, as slowly as the tempo set for the duration of the entire exercise, which for the beginner is twenty minutes. Even though, as a beginner, you will not be able to sustain an even tempo, you must nevertheless execute the action slowly. This slowness is so basically natural that you cannot but find the right tempo when you start, because the design, from the very first movement, leads you into the proper tempo, provided, of course, that you *think* in terms of moving slowly. Note that no mention has been made of music accompaniment because no outside stimulus is necessary for this intrinsic exercise. You yourself are in control; you *are* the tempo, the rhythm, the form, and the spirit. As one masters the exercise, the tempo can be slowed down and the total time increased to twenty-five or thirty minutes. When expert, you can, with unerring assurance, prolong the time as you wish, without losing the relationship of time, space, and form in exact synchronization.

There are many reasons for moving with slowness. Slowness aids in the process of developing awareness. You have more time to observe what you are doing, since you are doing half as much in twice the time. Patience and poise come with sustaining slow, physical control.

To be able to move slowly with conscious control dispels ill temper and irritability. When one is nervous, gestures are irregularly fast and staccato. Slow motion soothes the nerves. "To exercise slowly is to be light; to be light is to be calm." With slowness you can savor the movement. Aesthetically, you can appreciate the most delicate turn of the wrist as well as the intangible detail of a large design. You are sensitized to the dynamics of change, to intricacies of pattern, to the weaving of space. You can experience the moment of synchronized stillness and the dovetailing process of movement.

The purely physical power accumulated by means of this slow technique is a reservoir of energy. The ability to fix attention and gather strength develops quick reactions and reflexes. "If one can control slowness, then one can act speedily."

Lightness (Ch'ing)

This aspect of movement encompasses continuity, softness, regularity, evenness, smoothness and flow. The Chinese image, as it applies to these qualities, relates to a delicate, difficult, patience-demanding occupation—that of getting the silk out of a cocoon intact: "Manipulating outer energy is like pulling silk." To strain and pull is to break the thread. To force motion and to exert falsely put a strain on the system. To overdo is to break the thread, and to underdo is not to get it at all. To have lightness in T'ai Chi Ch'üan is to be able to draw out the movement uninterruptedly from beginning to end. This, like the silk, which has tensile strength, will give a sustained vitality with the power of long life.

To have lightness enables one to move flowingly. To move with flow is to be even and continuous; to be continuous is to be endless; to be endless one must move in curves; to move in curves is to be light.

Clarity (Chieh)

Referring expressly to the mind, this word clarity combines the concepts of clean and pure. If the mind can be concentrated on the process of action, it will be cleansed of intruding thoughts. I have taken the liberty of extending the concept of clarity to the physical aspect of the Forms. If the mind is purely directed, then the Forms will be cleanly done. If the Forms are made purely, cleansed of carelessness and inaccuracies, then the mind inevitably has clarity. With the mind alerted, no form can be vague, nor will the outline of movement be irregular, amorphous, ragged, or inexact. It is with clarity that the mind weaves a wholeness, since it is not merely a matter of doing but also of knowing.

Balance (Heng)

"Gravity is the root of grace, the mainstay of all speed" (by Lao-tzu, translated by Witter Bynner).

To be well balanced is to be in full control of both static and mobile equilibrium. Balance applies to the physical body and to a state of harmony that is emotional and mental. At every moment in the course of the patterned sequences there is complete and mathematical balance. T'ai Chi Ch'üan is unlike any other exercise in that it necessitates having or being in constant balance. When a body is in perfect balance, there is no strain on any part of it.

For balance one must necessarily have (1) physical ability, (2) an understanding of movement sequences, (3) an even flow of movement and the control of the inactive, (4) control of the changes from Yin to Yang and from Solid (Shih) to Empty (Hsü), (5) control of movement from space to form, (6) mental awareness, and (7) a spirit of calmness. All these requirements balance themselves and contribute to the mastery of each part. As gradually and imperceptibly as a root takes hold, as a plant grows, as a stem lengthens, and as flowers mature, so inevitably does balance become serenity. "When a master stands, he is in perfect balance and moves like a carriage wheel."

Calmness (Ching)

"Calmness is of decisive importance." You are asked to start with calmness and to make your mind direct the action. In a fraction of a second you can "suspend the torrents of thoughts" by this act of attentiveness. An even flowing continuity creates calmness. Smooth manipulation of movement sustains this sense of repose; and thus ease of mind grows out of form and technique. With the development of stability, both physical and mental, a state of calmness becomes habitual.

"Action—seek quiet inside," refers to a blending of action and quiet that affects the entire system. Action keeps one from getting too lax, and quietness keeps one from getting too hard.

The everchanging variety of Yin and Yang, in "peaceful" relationship, gives mental and bodily equilibrium; the structural integration of the Forms, being a work of art as well as a work of science, contains a natural harmony that is in itself calmness.

Without calmness there can be no concentration; without concentration there can be no co-ordination; and without co-ordination there is no harmony.

Slowness, lightness, clarity, balance, and calmness, softness, and circular movement are basic, and are united and interdependent, as are the Forms between which there are no gaps. Every movement is the instigator of what follows and the result of what has preceded. They are also like harmonious chords in music—simultaneously apparent—where each note responds to the overtones of the others and deeply influences the others' essence. As in the waveline of the T'ai Chi, they move in endless succession; and like its delineating circumference, these elements are fused, without beginning and without end. In T'ai Chi Ch'üan, whether one starts with the mind and continues with the body, or starts with the body and continues with the mind, there is always a state of harmony. "Gradual comprehension comes from growing familiarity which leads one to superlative clarity [mastery]." "But unless one pursues this exercise long enough he cannot hope to understand. . . because nothing can be mastered all of a sudden."

In this book I have incorporated technical ideas that have grown out of teaching situations, to give students not only an intellectual awareness of what T'ai Chi Ch'üan is, but also to create the understanding with which to experience its essence, as well as the physical form. We know too well that this process cannot be hurried unnaturally; nevertheless, the way can be illuminated by "quietly studying and analyzing [and then] one gradually by degrees learns to do the bidding of the mind."

"To go a thousand miles one has to take the first step" is a familiar Chinese saying. Each step, ostensibly, is like the following one, but the added experience that each brings to the next one contributes to endurance, agility, and strength. The act of self-study which by its very nature involves will power, thought, and awareness, is a dynamic step forward. The great variety of Forms and the intensely interesting techniques, the subtleties of which unfold with experience, and the sheer beauty of the postures, give delight, even if one has not mastered them, and keep one constantly alert and stimulated. To practice the exercise at any stage of one's development is to be better and to feel better.

As one develops understanding and progresses with the technique, T'ai Chi Ch'üan becomes a richer entity, seemingly limitless in what it has to offer. The ability to perform it for its minimum of twenty to twenty-five minutes gives one lasting good health. To perfect it and to live with it as a life-long exercise is to assure oneself of stable health, mental alertness, and equanimity of spirit.

PART II

FUNDAMENTALS

GENERAL REMARKS

Release yourself from the thought of time pressing in on you. The factor of time enters into the fact of progress. By doing, you begin to know. By knowing, you then begin to do.

The slower the exercise is done, the lighter it looks but the weightier it feels. Sensations of lightness and strength are simultaneous. Speeding up reveals plasticity; slowing down reveals form. However, for the observer, the form seems to be revealed by quick motion and the plasticity by slow movement. Each movement is like a drop of water in a moving stream; the beginning and the end cannot be seen. To maintain a flowing action, you must have control beneath the surface: the lighter and smoother it looks, the more muscular control it has.

To comprehend is to know mentally; to apprehend is to sense and feel. For T'ai Chi Ch'üan you must both know and feel. As a long exercise, it builds up energy gradually. As you grow with it, from two, to five, to ten, and finally to twenty minutes, you are never exhausted, because the development is natural, unstrained, easy, and inevitable.

Note the difference between the slow movement of T'ai Chi Ch'üan and the slow motion of a moving picture in which the action is made to move more slowly than is possible in real life, as for example in the artificial slow motion of a diver in space. In T'ai Chi Ch'üan, because the body is always in a state of equilibrium and the designs are related to each other in impeccable balance, the movement can be slowed down to an enormous degree, depending on the technique and control of the doer. This is *real* slow motion.

To make legs move in a perfectly flowing way, muscular stamina is needed. To make arms and torso move in a perfectly flowing way, it is not physical strength that is needed; it is concentration and awareness and conscious control.

With concentration there is stillness, in balance there is concentration, and in stillness there is balance. Equilibrium of body, heart, and mind makes one feel "at one with oneself."

"True quiet means keeping still when the time has come to keep still, and going forward when the time has come to go forward. In this way, rest and movement are in agreement . . . with the demands of the time. . . ." *I–Ching,* Book of Changes

PRINCIPLES TO BE OBSERVED

1. Always keep in mind: slowness, lightness, clarity, balance, and calmness.
2. Be consistent in tempo.
3. Fix attention on what you are doing at the moment you are doing it.
4. Remember: approach T'ai Chi Ch'üan from point of view of mind as well as body.
5. Movement is based on the normal, natural way the body functions: keep head straight, waist loose, buttocks in, joints open, and arms easy.
6. If you exercise for strength alone you will lose the spirit; if you exercise for spirit alone you will lose the Form and not achieve the proper spirit.
7. Each movement spurs on the next movement; this is continuous and flowing form.
8. Do not make your steps too small; they must be in correct proportion to your size.
9. You will acquire balance if you distinguish between the Empty and the Solid Steps.
10. Distinguish between the various hand positions: Yin, Yang, and Standing (neutral). Be aware of where the finger tips are directed.
11. Do not exert; do not use all your strength; you should move with springlike tension, capable of great expansion.

12. Distinguish between the active and the inactive parts of your body. One part of your body is in motion all the time, but not the same part.
13. That part of your body which is not in movement must be held firmly, but not rigidly, with conscious control.
14. The upper part of your body—torso and head—must be light. The lower part below the waist controls the weight and solidity. This is the proper body balance—otherwise you would be top-heavy, clumsy, and off-balance.
15. Motion follows a circular shape like that of the T'ai Chi symbol, in which there are different degrees of dynamics.
16. Keep the harmonious sequence of feet, knees, legs, waist, hand, and head.
17. Every movement has its counterpart: forward-backward, in-out, up-down, in opposition–together, right-left.
18. Strength comes from the hands, not from the forward pressure of the shoulders.
19. Every movement and every small fraction within it is of equal importance. Do not flourish the hand movements; the smaller the movements, the more difficult they are to control in proper tempo.
20. Note the *fast* movements well; these are difficult to do clearly and speedily. Keep in mind the reasons for these patterns: (1) they increase one's ability to move from a slow action to a quick one without external preparation; (2) they increase one's ability to recover one's basic tempo from a more rapid one without a transition; (3) they center the attention or bring back the attention, if one has been lulled by the slow, flowing movements; (4) and as my teacher Ma Yüeh-Liang laughingly said, "They keep you from getting bored!"
21. Remember: "Attention centers not on things in their state of being but upon their movements in change." *I—Ching*, Book of Changes

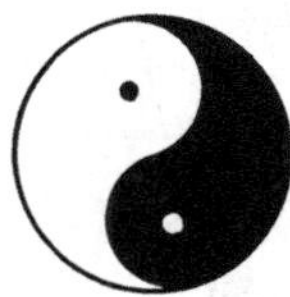

The T'AI CHI Symbol

It is necessary to familiarize yourself with the basic positions that are part of the technique of T'ai Chi Ch'üan. Knowing them well will facilitate the process of learning the Forms as a whole.

Use them as reference but do not utilize them as exercise. In the text itself, only, are they done as an exercise together with the movements that precede and follow them. The principle involving the interplay of Yin and Yang, and of "Empty and Solid," on which the exercise is based, will then not be violated.

1. Posture: You must stand straight and be centered (Chung); you should feel comfortable, easy (An Shu), without tension or strain. To achieve this natural, comfortable position, the head is held straight at "a ninety degree angle to the horizon," so that the top of the head is directed upward. The neck is held tall, lightly and "humbly"—this means without strain or tension, which is arrogant, and without limpness, which is submissive. (Figure 1, page 45)

Your shoulders must be low and loose, which frees both neck and back from tenseness. The chest is neither pushed up nor hollowed out. The abdomen must not protrude or be overcontracted.

The spine is straight but not stiffened, with buttocks not protruding. If body balance is correct, the hips will be even and level. An overarched spine is a stiff spine, which thrusts hips backward and throws the coccyx out of alignment.

No joint is stiffened or locked. The arms hang in their natural

Figure A

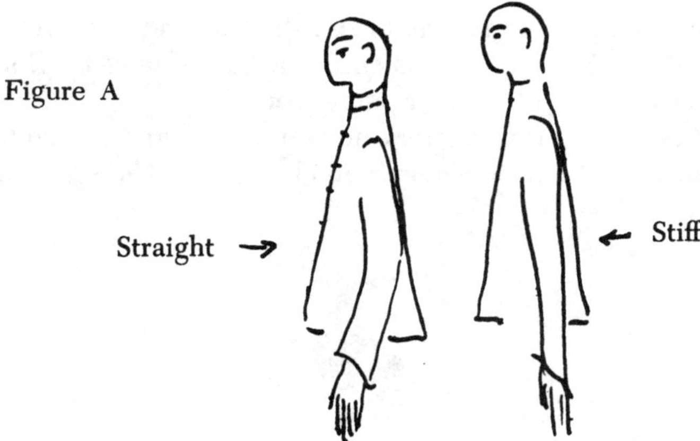

line with loose elbows. (Figure A) The legs are straight with knee joints flexible.

The torso should feel light. You should feel firm and supported solidly by the area below the waist and by the legs.

You should feel light "as if suspended by the top of the head," yet so strong that "you could support the world."

2. *Your Basic Stance* (P'ing Hsing Pu): Place your feet parallel and apart, separated by a distance equal to the length of your foot. Your feet are therefore, as it were, set on the sides of a square. "The feet are the earth and the head is heaven." (Figure B)

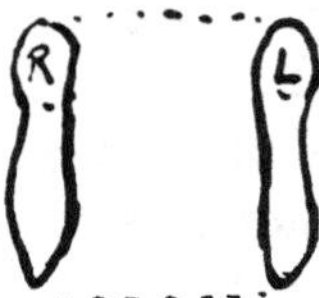

Figure B. Basic Stance (parallel and apart—a square)

3. *Bent-Knee position:* Take your stance with feet parallel and apart. Bend both knees equally; keep back straight as it is lowered by the bending of the knees. Feel the active movement at the waist, which must take place when you keep your spine straight and buttocks tucked under. (Figure 3, page 46)

Points of knees are directly over the toes; do *not* let knees pull together.

4. *Flexed Foot position, the Empty Step* (Hsü Pu): Take your basic stance with feet parallel and apart. Bend both knees equally. Then move left leg directly forward, raise toes upward, and touch heel to ground lightly. Straighten left knee. Your weight is on right leg with its bent knee. There is no weight on left leg. This is the Empty Step, which means that it is empty of any weight. (Figure 4, page 47)

The Solid Step (Shih Pu) is on that foot which holds the weight. To maintain perfect balance, the transition from Empty to Solid must be carefully controlled.

Each position may be made on either foot.

5. *Loose Foot position:* This is also an Empty Step. Take your basic stance. Bend both knees equally. (1) Then draw left foot close to right foot; let left foot hang loosely with toes resting lightly

on floor; left knee is bent. Weight is on right leg with its bent knee. Spine is straight. Do not stretch or extend the instep. Let the foot hang naturally. (Figure 68, page 93) (2) Raise left leg slightly; take toes off floor; keep toes close to right foot. This also is a Loose Foot position. This position occurs when a foot is in transition from one step to another. (Figure 25A, page 60)

6. *The T-Step position* (Ting-Tzu Pu) or *Toed-In Step:* Take your basic stance with feet parallel and apart. Now change to Empty Step position—bring left leg forward, flex foot, and touch left heel on floor, lightly; straighten left knee. From this Empty Step, turn left toes toward the east, or right, by pivoting on heel which remains on the same place on floor. Place left foot flat on floor, so that toes point to right, and it is at right angles to the right foot. Transfer weight onto left leg, and bend left knee, straightening right knee; keep right foot on floor (do not raise heel off floor). This is the T-step, or Toed-In Step. (Figure 6, page 48)

This position occurs on either foot.

7. *Seated position* or *Horse-Riding Step* (Ch'i Ma Pu): Separate your feet by a space equal to twice the length of your foot. Place your toes out at a *slight* angle. Bend both knees equally. Direct knees over toes. Keep back straight and buttocks under. Do not arch the back. Weight is equal on both legs. (Figure 13, page 53)

8. *The Walking Step position* or *Bow Step* (Kung Pu), and the *Walking Step Space:* Take your basic stance with feet parallel and apart facing west (or to the left side of the room). Now bring left leg forward in the Empty Step position (see Number 4), with left heel touching ground lightly; weight is on right leg with its bent knee. Now transfer weight onto left leg, placing entire foot flat on floor, and bend left knee at the same time. Straighten right knee keeping right heel on floor. Torso slants forward on a diagonal with body in a straight line from head to right heel; spine is straight and buttocks remain tucked under; hips are even; shoulders are

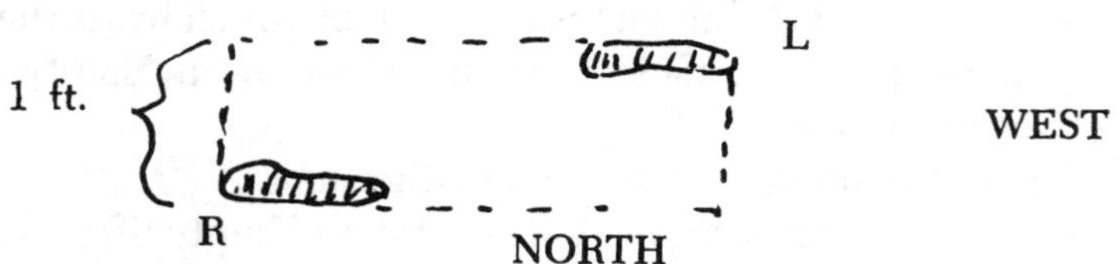

Figure C1. Toes are pointing west. This is the Walking Step Space. Feet are one foot apart, separated in length by one and a half feet, more or less.

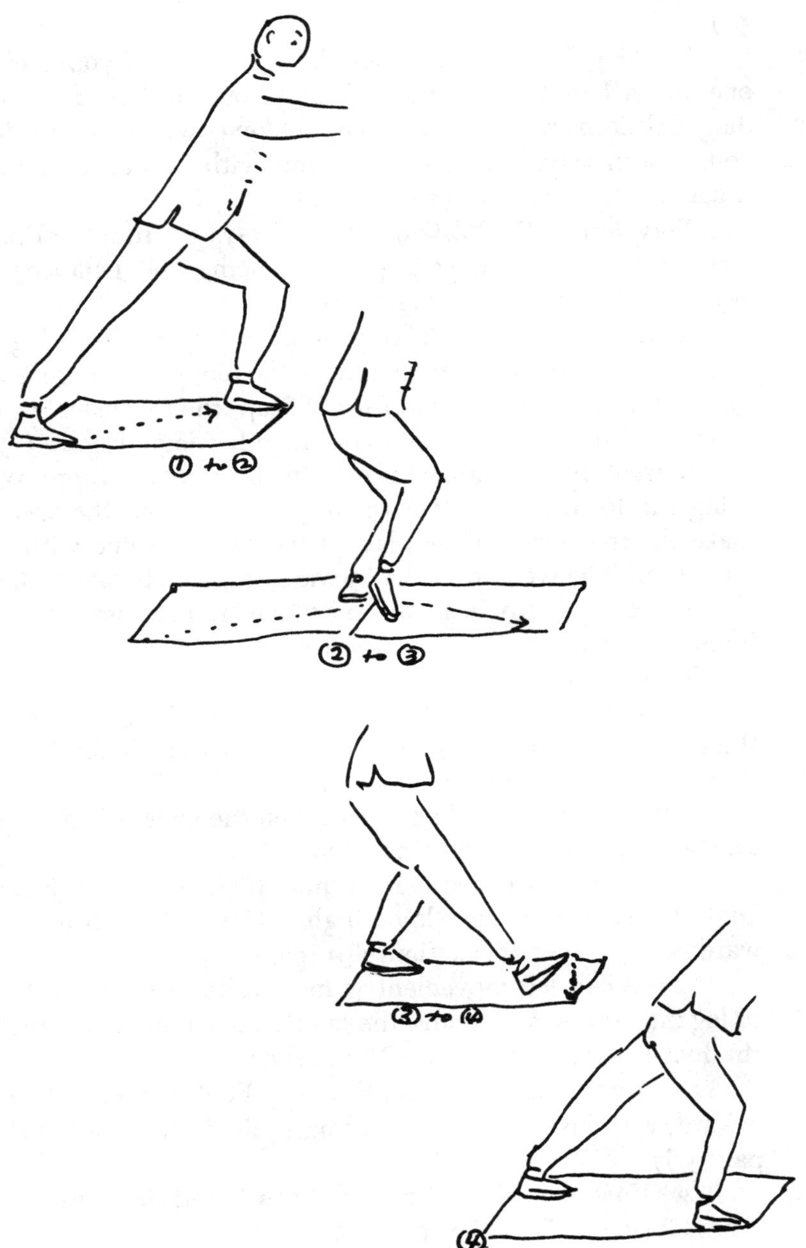

Figure C

even; the chest and abdomen are centered; and head remains in line with neck and shoulders (do not tilt it or drop it). (Figure 25, page 59)

Walking Step Space: Notice that the length of your step is about one and a half times the length of your foot. The feet are in the diagonal corners of an imaginary oblong, which is one length of your foot in width. Each foot is in line with its hip, so that the body is completely centered. (Figure C1)

Traveling in the Walking Step: always go from the Empty Step (from which you find your proper spacing and balance) into the Walking Step itself. (Figure C1 to 2)

Advancing in the Walking Step: Bring the back leg from its position, close to the other one: make the foot loose (Figure C2 to 3); then place it forward in the Empty Step; then transfer weight onto it. You are in the Walking Step on the other leg. (Figure C3 to 4, 4)

Retreating (going backward) in the Walking Step: When you bring the forward leg close to the one on which the weight rests, make the foot loose. Then place it backward in line with your hip; do not take the weight off the forward leg, which has all the weight.

The entire body is always on a slant in the completed Walking Step.

These positions occur on either side.

9. *Raised Leg position:* When a leg is raised and *straightened*, the knee must not be *stiffened*. The lower part of the leg is in line with the thigh. (Figure 72, page 96)

When a leg is raised and *bent*, then the knee is kept high. There are two examples for this position.

(1) When lower leg is held quite high, and thigh is held at an angle to body with bent knee high. (The foot is always flexed inward, see Number 10.) (Figure 91, page 109)

(2) When leg movement is in transition; then the lower part of leg moves downward and the knee bends at an acute angle, while the foot is always loose (see Number 5).

10. *Foot position* (Chiao Fa): (1) Foot is extended and turned inward, with instep and *toes* leading (called T'i Chiao). (Figure 72, page 96)

(2) Foot is flexed and turned inward, with *heel* leading (called Teng Chiao). (Figure 91, page 109)

11. *Movements of Feet—Toes and Heel:* Take your basic stance with feet parallel and apart with knees bent. Pivoting on right

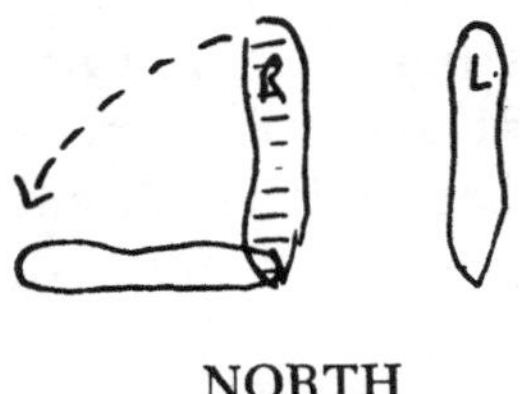

NORTH

Figure D. The shaded foot is the moving foot.

toes, move right heel to the right. Straighten left knee. Keep right knee bent; try not to show shift of weight. Your torso is turned to west. You are now in a T-Step, with toed-in position. This occurs on either foot. (Figure D)

Take the Seated Position (as in Number 7) with feet apart twice the length of your foot and toes out at a slight angle. Turn right toe inward slightly, making right foot parallel to left foot; then move right heel outward, getting into a T-Step or toed-in position. Keep right knee bent with weight on it. Straighten left knee. This occurs on either foot. There are always *two* movements on one foot, when the foot moves from a seated position. (Figure E1, Figure E2)

12. *The Toe-Heel-Heel Step:* This is a combination of the T-Step and your basic stance with feet parallel and apart. Take the Walking Step position with left leg forward, left knee bent, body

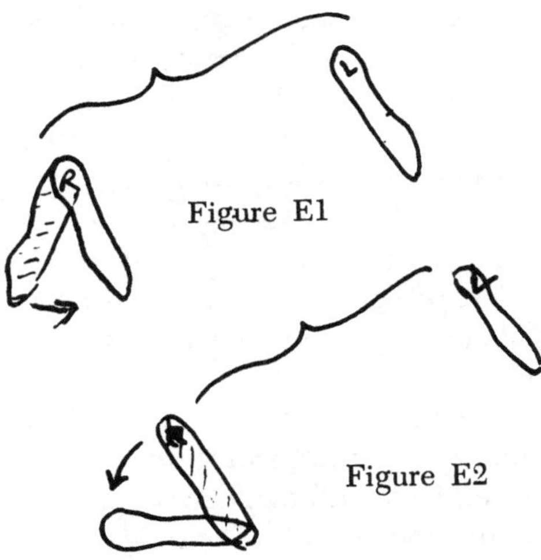

Figure E1

Figure E2

slanting forward, right leg straight. Turn left toes inward, keep weight on left leg with its bent knee, straighten hips out so that torso is erect. Then move right heel inward and bend right knee; weight is still on the left side. This movement makes the feet parallel. Now move left heel outward keeping weight on left leg with its bent knee; straighten right knee, and now you are in the T-step on the other side.

From this step move into the Empty Step: with weight on left leg with its bent knee, raise right toes and keep right heel lightly on ground; foot is flexed, and knee is straight. Feet are parallel, although right foot is flexed (otherwise right foot would be in toed-in position). You are seated on left with bent knee. (Figure 39, page 69)

Level of body must be kept even during these changes.

This step is only done from left to right; weight remains on left during movement.

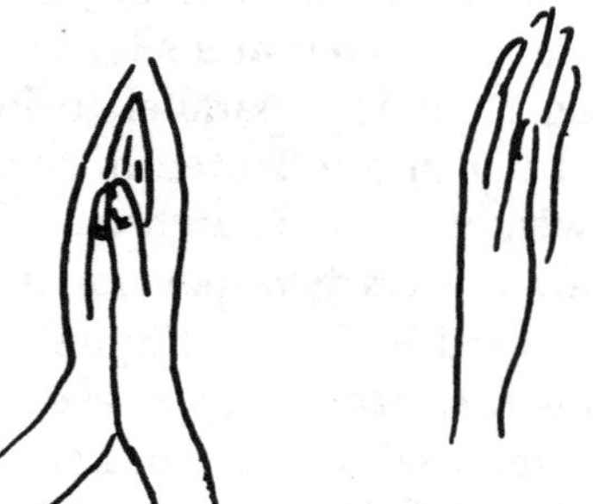

Figure F

13. *The Hand position* or *Palm method* (Chang Fa) and *the Hand Form:* The hands are held loosely, knuckles and joints are not stiffened or tightened. From the position where your arms hang down, with loose elbows, note the hand form. The hands curve inward slightly, and the palm is curved. (Figure F)

Hands facing outside or away from body or upward are Yang. (Figure 25, page 59) Hands facing inward or toward body or downward are Yin. (Left hand, Figure 5, page 47) When palm faces to right or left of body, with fingers forward or upward, it is called Standing Palm (with an element of Yin). (Right hand, Figure 72, page 96)

14. *The Fist position* (Ch'üan Fa): Close fingers not too tightly. Fold thumb over second and third fingers. Wrist is generally straight with a fisted hand. Elbows are dropped, that is, they point downward in a punch movement. (Figure 30, page 63)

15. *The Finger position:* Fingers are generally held rather close together. In some forms the fingers are spread wide and apart from each other. (Figure 71, page 95) There is one special position, the Paw (Chua) or Grasping position, where finger tips are close together grasping the thumb. The tip of the thumb touches the fingers at their base. Wrist is bent and the hand knuckles are bent. In this position, fingers always point to the floor. Finger tips must be directed correctly toward positions (concentration of energy in tips). (Right hand, Figure 13, page 53)

16. *The Wrist position:* (1) Wrists are straightened so that hand and arms make a straight line. (Figure 36, page 67) (2) Wrists are bent so that hand can face in many directions, at right angles to arm (Figure 25, page 59) (3) Wrists bend sideways: stretch arm forward with hand facing inward; move hand so that finger tips point diagonally downward, or diagonally upward; this is bending the wrist sideways. (Figure 28, page 62)

17. *Shoulder and Elbow position:* The shoulders must be controlled so that they do not push the movement; all strength comes from spine, not shoulders. Shoulders must be kept in *place,* not forward or pulled up. The elbows are kept low. When shoulders are loose and low, it is possible to control arm movement. When elbows are pointed outward or raised out of their natural position, then the shoulders are pulled forward out of place. (Figure 7, page 49, and Figure 33, page 65)

18. *Waist position:* The waist is an important hinge, which must be loose and relaxed, but not slack. You must not press down into it. The torso lifts up from it. It is as "active as a cartwheel." When the waist can turn, the spine is flexible. The waist and spine control the exact position of the coccyx. If correct, they pull the buttocks in; when stiff, the back goes out "like a mountain peak." Hips must be kept level. (Figure 34, page 65)

19. *Eyes:* The eyes, unless directed to move with the hands, look diagonally forward (in relation to where the head is) with a quiet, easy, but steady gaze. "The eye is the cottage of the spirit."

20. *Mouth and Tongue position:* Mouth must be kept lightly shut. The tip of tongue touches upper palate, behind teeth. The mouth is thus kept moist. "Saliva is sweet dew for cultivating life."

21. *Breathing:* Breathe naturally, through the nose. The Forms will make you breathe deeply at certain times. Breathing is always regular in tempo.

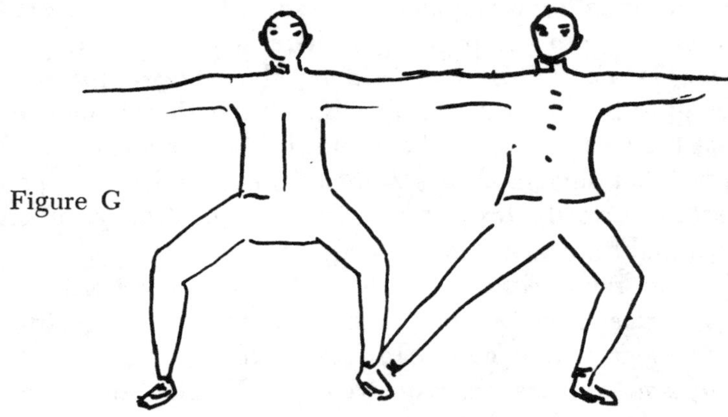

Figure G

22. *Body:* The body must be held "as steady as a mountain," and must feel "as light as a bird's feather."

23. *Stepping position:* The steps must be evenly paced and rhythmically exact as is "the walk of a cat." The toes of the forward foot must be directed exactly toward the angle of the designated design; for example, on stepping in the Walking Step toward the west, the toes of the forward foot must point exactly west.

24. *Shifting of Weight:* In the process of shifting your weight from one leg to the other, you must move so that the level of the head (torso and hips) remains the same. In changing position from one leg which is bent, to the other leg which is straight, the action is smooth and flowing. This is done by controlling the knee bends. (Figure G)

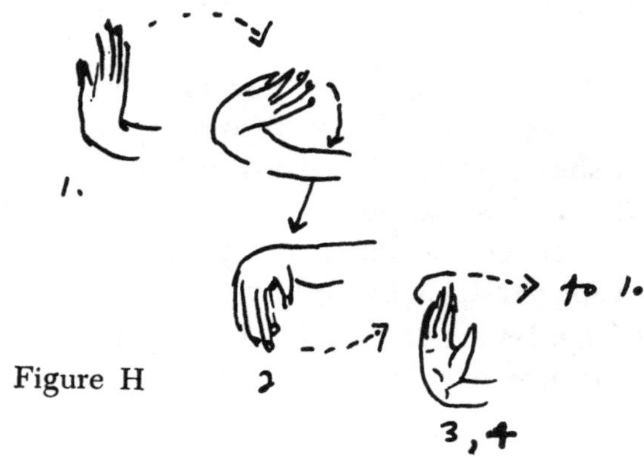

Figure H

25. *Hand Circling and Wrist Rotation:* The circles, or parts of circles, that the hands describe in some of the movements are an extremely important element in the consideration of T'ai Chi Ch'üan as a circular exercise. (1) Raise right arm forward shoulder high, with loose elbow, and bend wrist, pointing fingers upward with palm facing outward. (2) Circle hand outward to right; then bend hand downward making palm face inward. (3) Then circle over to the left and then upward with palm still facing inward, so that fingers point upward. (4) Turn palm outward, and it is once again in the starting position. Try to keep arm still, while the hand is moving. Do these movements with the left hand. Then circle both hands at the same time. Reverse the circle, making an inward rotation. (Figure H)

26. *Basic Tempo, Variations, and Synchronized Movements:* Control of tempo is essential for the proper synchronization of the Forms and patterns. The tempo with which you start the exercise is the basic one, the first movement of Form 1. When there is a variation, it is always *slower* than the basic tempo. In many Forms the arms will have to arrive at a given position at the same moment, although one may have to cover a larger space. Example: Raise your left arm forward, shoulder high, and raise your right arm up vertically. Both arms are to arrive at a low position along your side at the same moment. The right arm has farther to go, move it downward in the basic tempo. The left arm has a smaller space to travel, it therefore must move more slowly. This principle always holds: slow up the movement which has less space to traverse and must arrive at a given position, to coincide with a movement which has a greater distance to go.

27. *The Essence of the Motion:* The quality of the movement must never be strained. It is the control of movement, not the extent to which it can go, that gives both strength and softness at the same time.

28. *A Reserve of Energy:* The energy used must never be excessive or deficient; the first exhausts and the second delays development. In the process of learning, it is better to *underdo* than overdo. With properly guided energy you can feel "held together" and light at the same time. In action never strain at the joints. At every moment in the exercise you must have a reserve of energy and of movement which you know can be expanded at any moment.

PART III

PRELIMINARIES

SUGGESTIONS FOR STUDY

1. Read the directions out loud before you study each new sequence, but do *not* talk while you move. Let your mind direct you, so that you anticipate each movement as you act on it.
2. Give yourself enough time to learn and to practice. Try to do the exercise regularly each day. Do not do too much at one time.
3. Each section carefully done will contribute to your well-being. You will never be impatient if you keep this in mind.
4. You must proceed slowly and accurately. Learn, relearn, and check what you do. When you practice, do everything three times: (1) to learn; (2) to correct and remember; and (3) which is very important, to experience the unity of what you do, and to capture its spirit.
5. Even when you have to stop in order to remember a sequence, try to hold the movement suspended, not frozen, as if you were a suddenly stopped motion picture.
6. If you remember that a light, even, flowing movement is essential for the feeling of calmness, you will more easily attain it. The idea of calmness will give you smooth movement; the smooth movement will give you calmness. Also remember that the Forms and patterns themselves, weaving into each other as they do structurally, will develop this essential quality, make you acquire it, since form and its function (of tranquillity) are inextricably one.

7. Each time you start to practice, stand quietly for a few seconds. Fix your gaze steadily and lightly on the floor, at least ten feet away. Think of a slowly flowing river. This helps to eliminate outside problems and thoughts, and puts you in the mood for study.
8. Divide the units into parts; study each separately. Always organize the parts into their larger units and practice them as a flowing sequence. Distinguish between simultaneous and consecutive action. Do not omit the smaller details, such as moving a heel, toe, or hand, as each must be considered as a movement, complete in itself and as necessary to the structure as is the smallest part of a piece of complicated machinery.
9. Do not overwork a tiny part. Each unit must contain a light and strong movement; a leg, arm, and body movement, so that you benefit at each practice session from the activity of exercising the entire body.
10. Do everything lightly and without anxiety. Do not confuse lack of anxiety with lack of effort or industriousness. You must make an effort to direct yourself with will. Light in action and deep in mind will result from effort with understanding.
11. Don't be hasty. Move slowly. No matter how much effort you put into practicing, you will feel enriched because of the vital Forms and the easy, calm process of the movement.
12. Refer to Basic Positions frequently.
13. Associate the names of the Forms with the patterns that go with them. You will then understand how complete a unit each Form is; how the Yin-Yang elements are balanced; how the Solid and Empty are dynamically related to each other; how the structural themes merge; and how they vary. You will begin to comprehend the subtlety of the whole composition mentally, physically, and aesthetically.
14. Notice: (1) how you warm up gradually; (2) how you develop strength and power as you practice; (3) that your breathing remains quiet and easy; (4) that the heart beat is not accelerated; (5) that you can maintain an easy calmness while learning; (6) that when you complete your daily practice, you have a sensation of well-being and tranquillity.

EXPLANATORY NOTES

1. Space Directions: Directions are given in terms of the compass: north, east, south, west, and the diagonals northeast, northwest, southeast, southwest. This method simplifies the delineation of space and keeps the text clear as to the difference between the sides of the body (right, left, front, back) and the sides of space.

Facing the North Star, you know that east is at your right, west at your left, and south behind you. This same principle is used for the directions of the spatial patterns, except that here we disregard the sun's true directions. You must consider north that side of your room toward which you face to begin the exercise; then east is the right side of the room, west is the left side, and south is the back wall.*

The illustrations are drawn with north as the point of reference. Look at them as you look at a photographic image. Therefore north is at the lower side of the diagram, toward which you face to begin. It will not be difficult to orient yourself to this concept of space. When you are actually in action, you feel the directions at eye level.

The floor pattern in space (the movement of the feet) is designed so as to cover more space toward the west than toward the east of the starting point position. In the diagram, the dotted lines indicate the limit of space that you will traverse when you do the complete exercise. Therefore note the starting position (the arrow pointing north), which is at the east of the center of your room.

The exercise ends in exactly the same place at which it begins.

2. Names of Forms: It is necessary to keep the standard names of the Forms, even though their meaning in English seems obscure. Though the names are not consistent as to motivation, they all have significance. Some are technically graphic and describe physical movement, as does Brush Knee Twist Step. Some indicate what the movement is, as rendered in Self-Defense, as in Parry, Obstruct, Punch. Others are derived from concepts or associations (but are not pantomimic). These, as in Hand Strums the Lute, suggest that the movement is like that of the particular image named.

There are some that have metaphysical significance such as Seven Stars, which may refer to the Big Dipper or, as some believe,

* The above space directions with North as the front I have changed from the original Chinese way, which has South as the front.

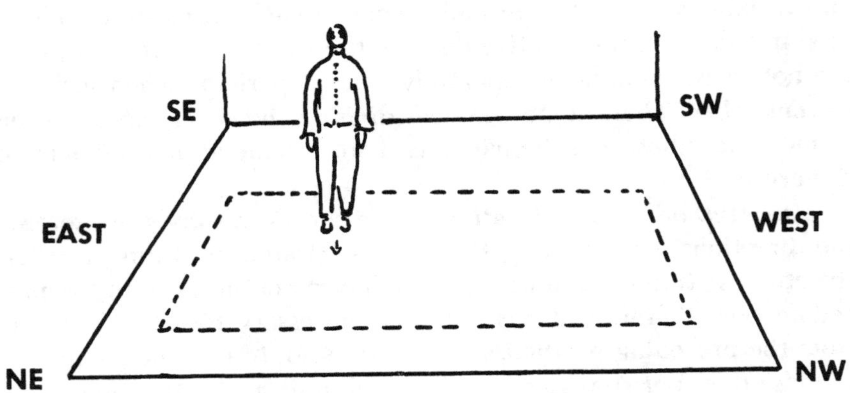

Space-Directions

to the seven openings of the head and heart. The Bird and Snake imply wit and intelligence.

Other terms are metaphorical, as in Carry Tiger, Push Mountain; the tiger stands for lungs, or respiration, and is Yin in quality. Perhaps The Stork Flaps Its Wings is so named because the movement activates that part of the body known as the Dove's Tail in ancient times. (It is an inch below the apex of the ensiform cartilage.)

For our purposes it is best to accept the names as terms with which to identify the various structures. It is necessary to remember them in order to appreciate the composition as a whole, and eventually to understand their significance as they relate to movement.

3. *Division into Series (I–VI):* Although the division of the 108 Forms into six series has been made to simplify the process of learning, it has not been done arbitrarily. Each series has structural meaning, as well as physical and psychological aspects. The developments and variations in the designs and themes of each series are distinctly vital in balancing the creative unity of the whole. Nevertheless, they are not to be thought of separately, except perhaps when learning to remember. There is no physical division, however, no cessation of movement between the parts, as there is none at any moment of the exercise.

4. *Method of Classification:* Since the Forms *are* the exercise, the directions for executing them are separated according to their structure. It is to be assumed that each part continues from the preceding one; therefore it has not been necessary to say, "Continue from the preceding position," each time. And, to reiterate, since the exercise does not stop at any point, each unit, no matter how small or large, is linked to the next one.

There are consecutive and simultaneous movements. And there are places where parts of the body are inactive, when other parts are active. Necessarily, the written directions have to isolate the various movements. Generally speaking, a complete part is described, with the legs', arms' and body's actions analyzed in a single paragraph. "At the same time," "simultaneously" indicate the synchronized action of several parts of the body. Unless otherwise stated, the action is consecutive; or if not mentioned at all, quiescence of the unmentioned part is to be assumed. These are to be carefully watched: stillness and movement, and consecutive and simultaneous action. The ultimate harmony of T'ai Chi Ch'üan lies in the relationship of consecutive flowing movement, the fleeting second of simultaneous completeness of movement, and the utter immovability of that part which must be quiet.

PART IV
THE PRACTICE OF T'AI CHI CH'ÜAN

SERIES 1

Form 1. Beginning Form of T'ai Chi Ch'üan

T'AI CHI CH'UAN CH'I SHIH

Face north. Stand tall, with head straight and shoulders low. With feet remaining parallel, separate them so that the space between them is equal to the length of your foot. This is your basic stance: feet parallel and apart. Your legs are on a perfect perpendicular. Place your arms down along your sides, with wrists straight and palms facing the rear (south). Look ahead of you on the floor about ten feet away. Feel centered, easy, quiet. Mouth is shut lightly, not tightly, and must remain so throughout the entire exercise. (Figure 1)

Raise both arms forward and up to shoulder level; wrists remain straight and are shoulder width apart. This simple movement establishes the tempo that you must maintain throughout the exercise; it focuses your mind and makes you feel light and calm. (Figure 1–A)

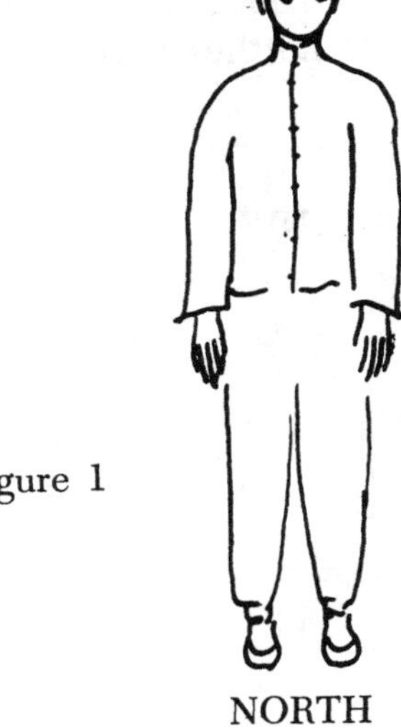

Figure 1

NORTH

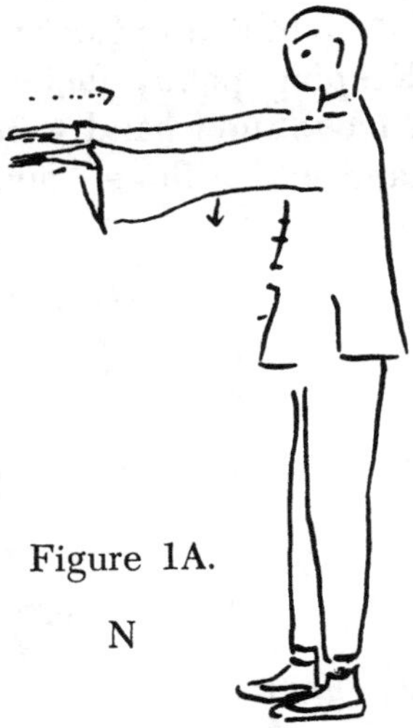

Figure 1A.

N

Side view from west

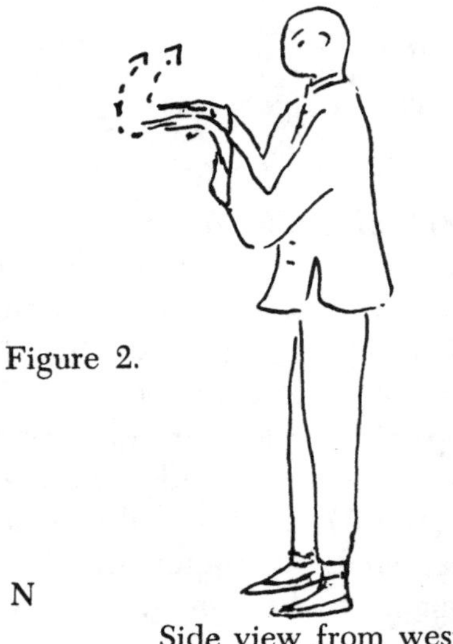

Figure 2.

Side view from west

Draw arms in toward shoulders by bending both elbows downward and slightly out, bending the wrists at the same time. Palms face the floor and are at shoulder height. (Figure 2)

Lift both hands so that they face north. Then move arms downward to the sides of thighs, keeping wrists bent with palms facing floor. At the same time as the arms move, bend both knees, keeping back straight and buttocks tucked in. (Figure 3)

Keeping palms facing floor, move both hands at the same time: move right hand so that fingers point to northeast, and move left hand so that fingers point to northwest.

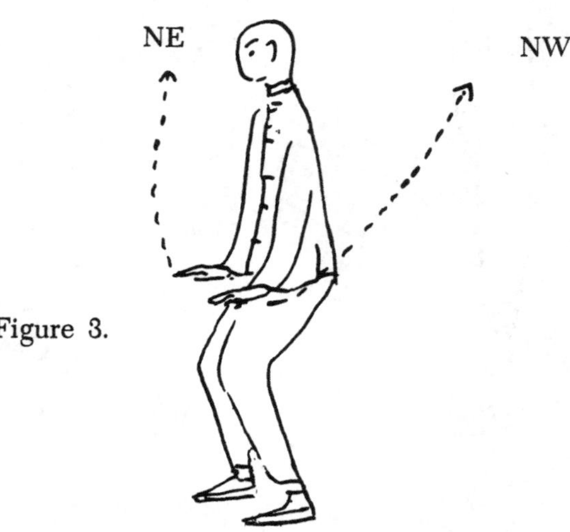

Figure 3.

Side view from west

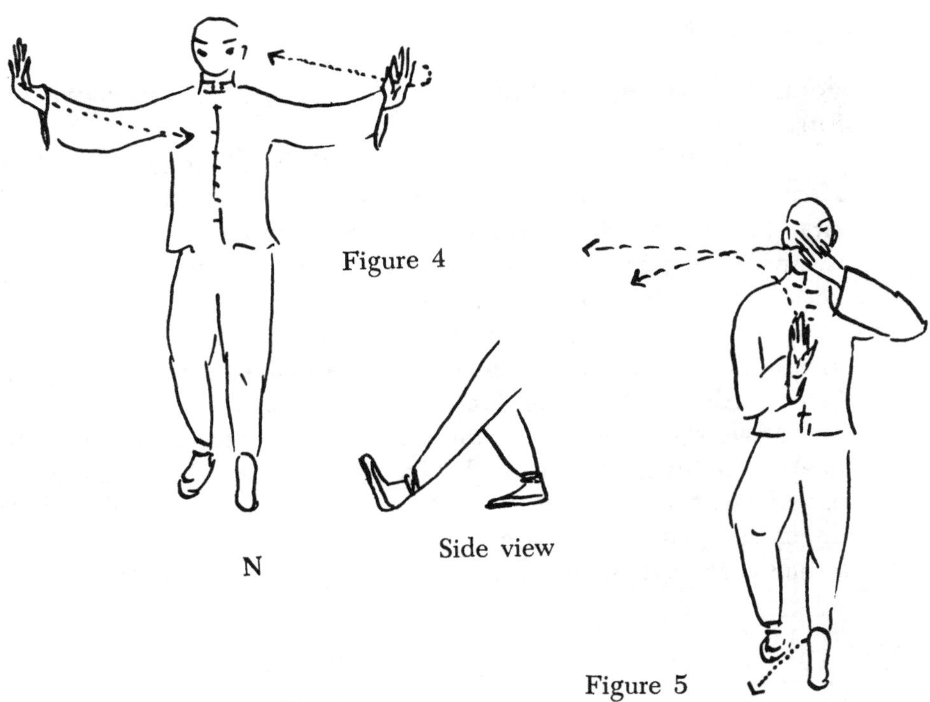

Figure 4

Figure 5

Raise both arms straight up in their diagonals, with fingers pointing upward. Right palm faces northeast and left faces northwest; both wrists come to slightly higher than shoulder level. At the same time as arms move, move left leg directly north, shifting all your weight onto the right leg with its already bent knee. Straighten left knee and place heel lightly on floor with toes upraised—this is a flexed foot (See page 27). Arms and legs arrive in position together. (Figure 4)

Hold this leg position (called Empty Step, see page 27). Both arms move at the same time: move right arm, with palm facing outward, to the center in front of chest about six inches away; turn left palm inward, moving arm to the front so that palm is toward the face and about twelve inches away. Left elbow is at about shoulder height; right elbows points side-downward. (Figure 5)

Form 2. Grasping the Bird's Tail LAN CH'UEH WEI

First

Turn toes of left foot toward the east, by pivoting on the heel. Place left foot on floor and bend knee at the same time, while straightening out the right knee. Weight is on the left leg and torso is turned to northeast. Feet are in the T-step position (see page 29) with left toes pointing east and right toes north.

As you place left toes to the east move both arms. Right arm moves to the east, left arm lowers to shoulder level, right palm faces north, and left palm faces south. (Figure 6)

Move right leg toward the east, straightening knee, and place heel on floor with foot flexed. Weight is on left leg. At the same time extend right arm to the east so that its pulse is at the point of left finger tips. Both elbows are loose and curved downward. Hands are at face level. Left fingers do *not* touch right pulse. (Figure 7)

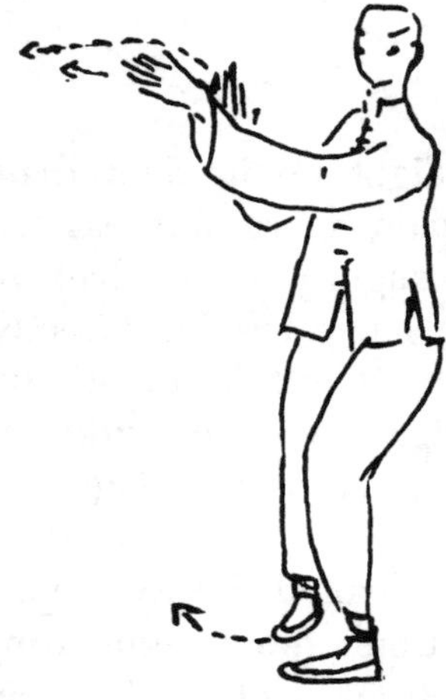

Figure 6

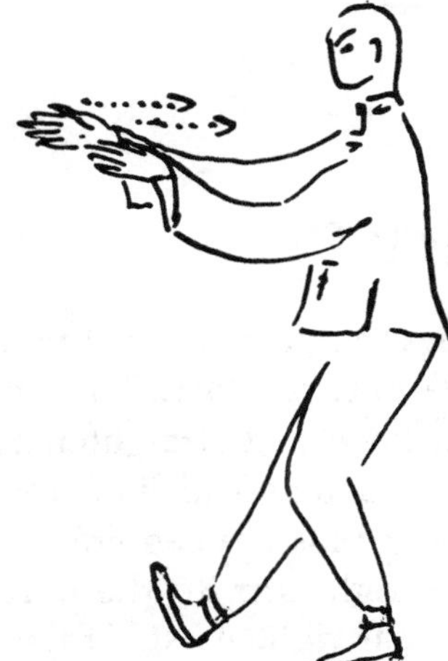

Figure 7

Keeping the relationship of hands the same, draw both arms in toward body at chin level, bending both elbows downward and slightly out. Do not come too close to face. Do not move legs.

Turn right palm up and left palm down. As you move hands, angle left hand so that it is at a right angle to right wrist; now left elbow points north. (Figure 8)

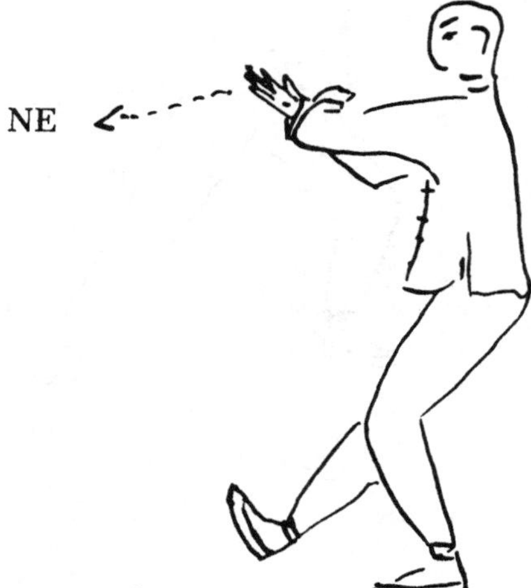

Figure 8

Form 3. Grasping the Bird's Tail **LAN CH'ÜEH WEI**

Second

Move right leg with straight knee in the Walking Step Space (see page 30) and place heel on floor. Then transfer weight onto right foot, bending right knee and straightening left knee. Weight is forward and body is on a diagonal line from head to left heel. Buttocks are tucked in and hips are centered. At the same time as you step forward, stretch right arm to the northeast, straightening elbow. Keep left fingers near right wrist. (Figure 9)

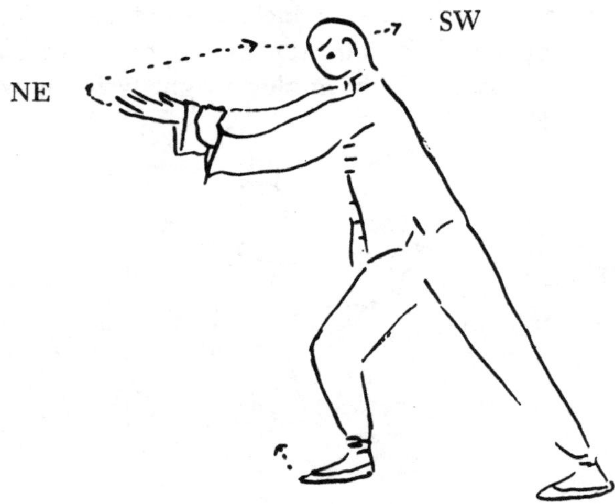

Figure 9

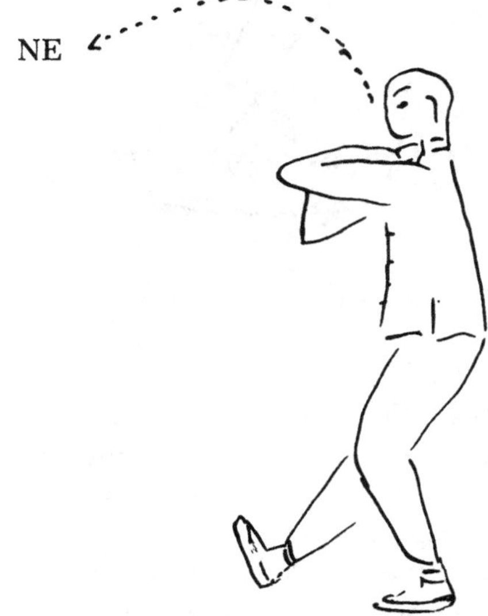

Figure 10

Circle both arms horizontally, chin high, going from northeast to east, to south, to southwest. When arms reach south, bend right elbow downward, bending right wrist so that palm faces upward toward ceiling. Both left and right fingers point southwest at the end of this horizontal circling. Left arm is adjusted to the movement of right arm, because left finger tips always remain near right pulse. (Figure 10)

At the same time as you are circling arms from south to southwest, shift weight back onto left leg by bending its knee, and straighten right leg, flexing right foot. (Figure 10)

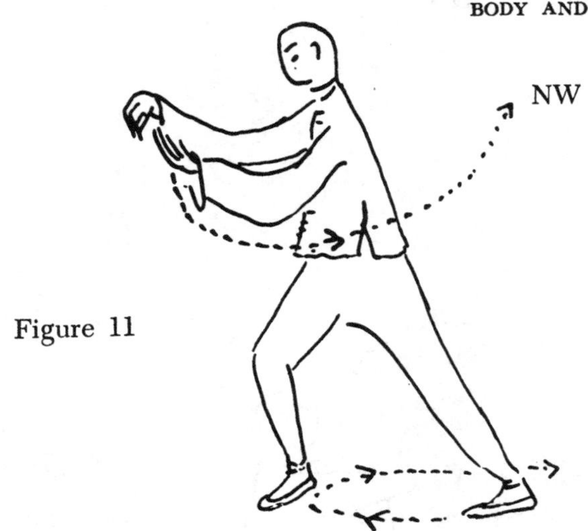

Figure 11

Form 4. Grasping the Bird's Tail LAN CH'ÜEH WEI
Third

Pivoting on right heel, turn right toes to northeast and place foot on floor. At the same time, raise right arm, with palm leading, up toward ceiling and circle it over and down toward the northeast, straightening arm as you do so. Stop in position when right wrist is slightly above shoulder height. (Figure 11)

As you are approaching this last position with the right arm, bend right knee, placing weight on right leg, and straighten left knee. At the same time, bend right wrist and lower hand, making fingers point downward. As hand bends down, place all the fingers over the thumb (Paw Hand) in grasping position (see page 32). Right arm does not move out of its position as hand bends down. Left fingers remain near right pulse with palm facing your face; left wrist is straight and arm is curved. (Figure 11)

Form 5. The Single Whip TAN PIEN

Hold weight on right leg with its bent knee. Draw left foot with loose ankle close to right, without touching floor with left toes. Then move left leg backward to southwest diagonal in the Walking Step Space (see page 30). Straighten left knee and place foot parallel to right foot; each foot is in its own track as in the Walking Step. Weight is on right leg, and body is on a diagonal slant toward northeast. As left leg moves, move left arm, with palm toward your face, in a downward curve in toward the body, waist high. Then raise it up and out toward the northwest, shoulder-high. Right arm does not move. (Figure 12)

Pivoting on left heel, turn toes toward the northwest. Place weight on left leg and bend knee to equal bend of right knee. Now your weight is even on both legs. Body is turned to northwest. Feet are separated by a distance equal to twice the length of your foot. Your back is straight. As left foot moves, turn left palm to face northwest, with fingers pointing upward. Now both arms are on the same level, with wrists slightly higher than shoulder level. Right arm is extended toward northeast, and left arm toward northwest; right toes point to northeast, and left toes to northwest. Right hand is in grasping position, and left wrist is bent with palm northwest. (Figure 13)

Movements of Head and Eyes for Form 5.

Take position as in Figure 11. Look at left palm; keep looking at it as hand moves down, and then up to northwest. Turn head from right to left side, but do *not* bend it downward when eyes look downward. The top of head is kept level as head moves from right to left side. When left palm turns to northwest, you will then be looking at the back of hand. (Figures 12 and 13)

Eyes, arm, legs, and body movements are synchronized.

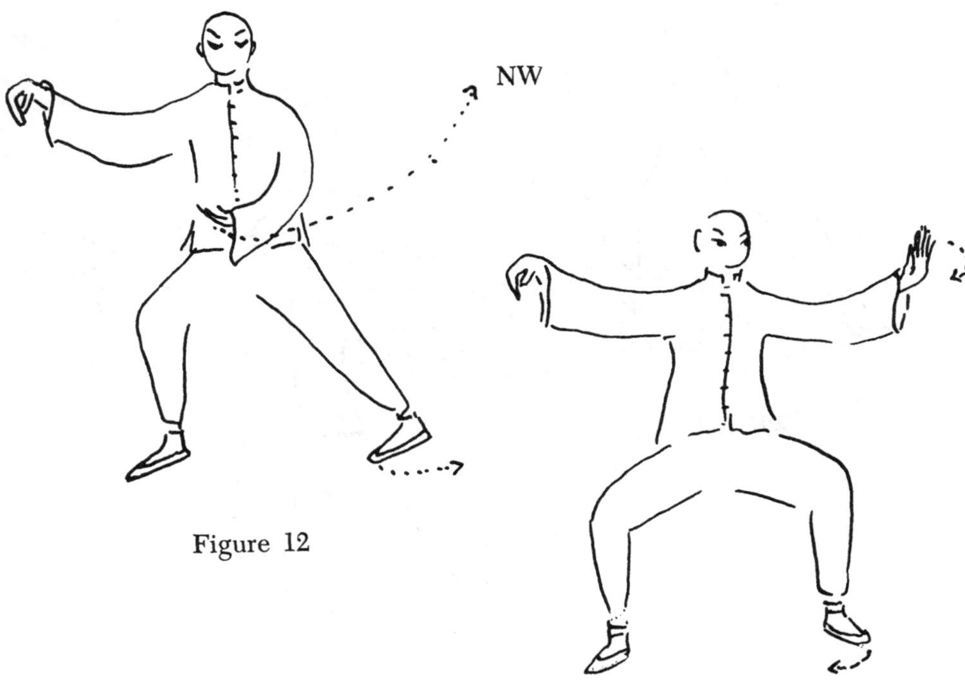

Figure 12

Figure 13

Form 6. Raise Hands and Step Up T'I SHOU SHANG SHIH

Keeping weight on left leg with its bent knee, turn toes of left foot to north and straighten right knee. At the same time, turn left palm upward, straightening wrist; fingers point to northwest. You are now looking at left palm. Do not tilt torso. (Figure 14)

Bend head so that left ear is directed toward left shoulder. Now the face is north, on a slant, with chin centered. As the head bends, open right hand and turn palm upward. Look at right palm, but do not move head. You are now looking obliquely toward the right. Right fingers point northeast. (Figure 15)

Turn right toes north. Bend right knee and straighten left leg. Place weight forward on right leg, lower torso, with rounded back, forward over right leg. Move both arms on this movement. Bring right arm in a curve forward, shoulder high, fifteen inches from

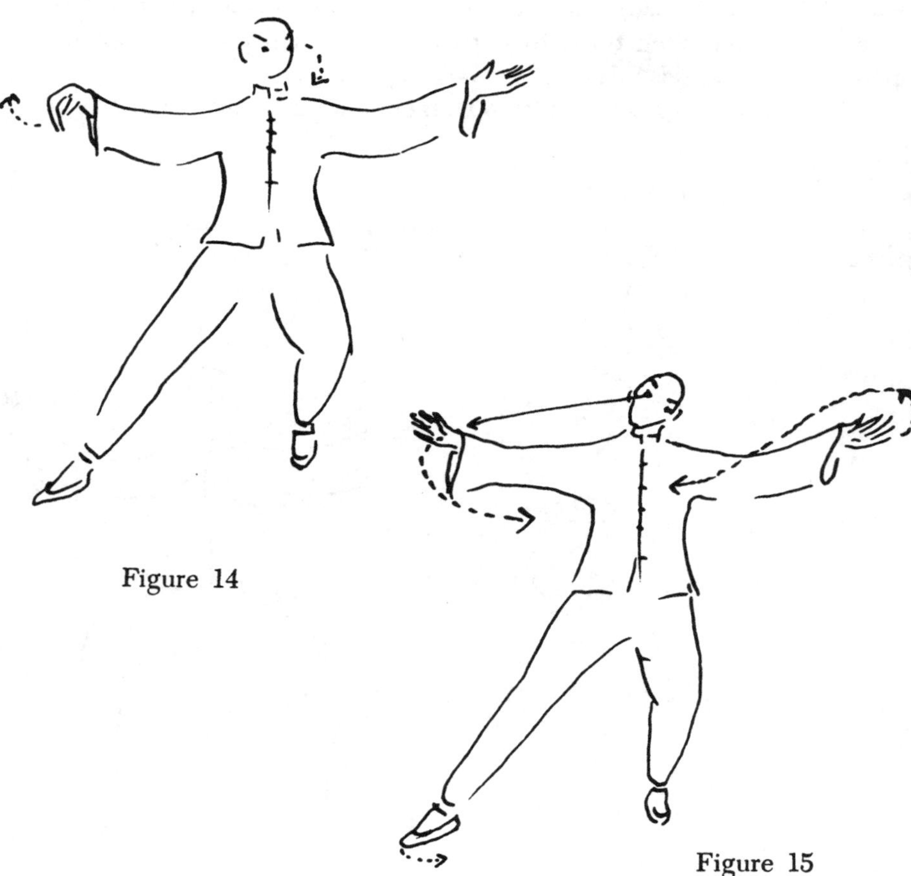

Figure 14

Figure 15

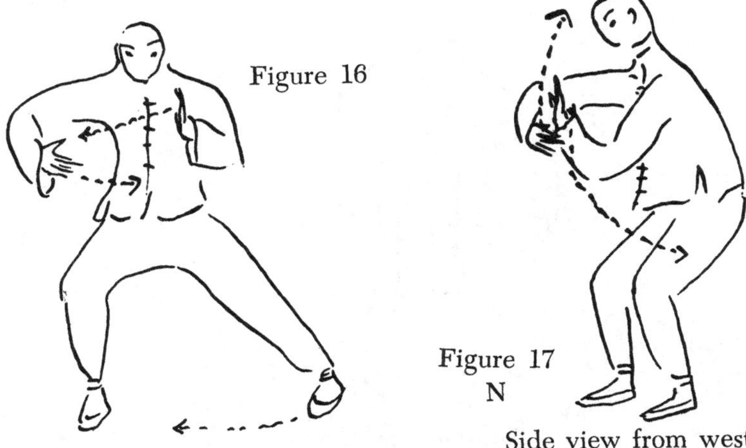

Figure 16

Figure 17
N
Side view from west

body, and move left hand, with palm turned toward northeast, directly to inner curve of the right elbow. Left elbow points downward, right elbow is shoulder high. (Figure 16)

Place left foot parallel and apart from the right foot, in your basic stance (Figure 1), bending left knee. Now both knees are evenly bent. The back is curved forward and weight is equal on both legs. (Figure 17)

Raise body to an upright position and straighten knees. At the same time, lift right curved arm to a position just above forehead, and lower left arm with palm down to front of left thigh. Wrist is bent and fingers point north. Arms and body finish together. (Figure 18) Then, as a separate movement, turn the right hand to face palm upward.

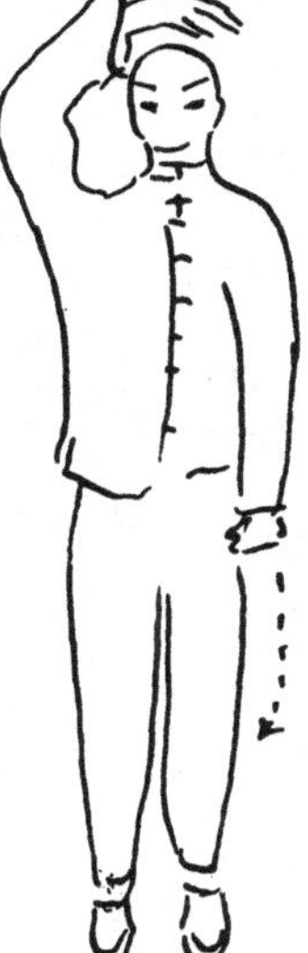

Figure 18

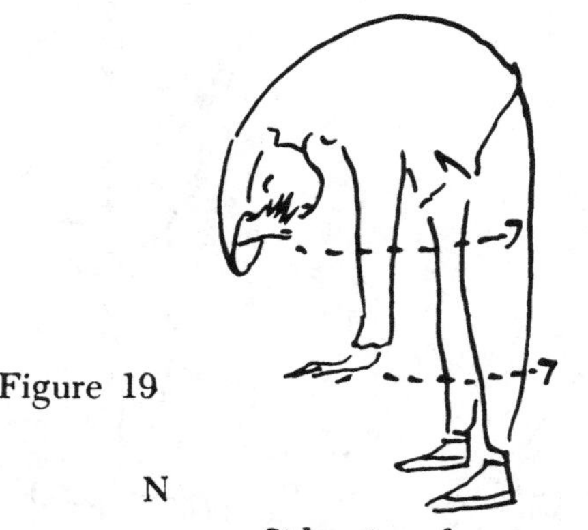

Figure 19

N

Side view from west

Form 7. White Stork Flaps Its Wings PAI HAO LIANG CH'IH

Do not move right arm from its place above forehead for the next sequences.

Bend torso forward down, and, at the same time, move left arm away from thigh so that it is perpendicular to floor, palm facing floor. (Figure 19)

Keep arms in same relative positions. Twist torso to west, keeping body low. Arms move with body. Fingers of left hand point west. (Figure 20)

Lift torso up erect, remaining turned to west. At the same time bring straight left arm up shoulder high. Left wrist is bent; palm faces west with fingers pointing upward. Head and torso are turned west; knees are straight. (Figure 21)

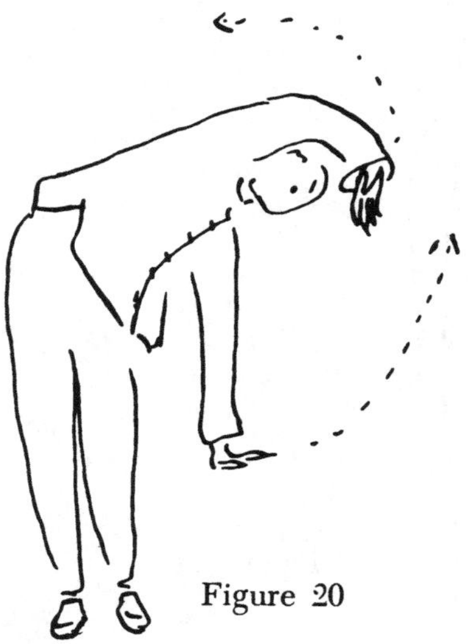

Figure 20

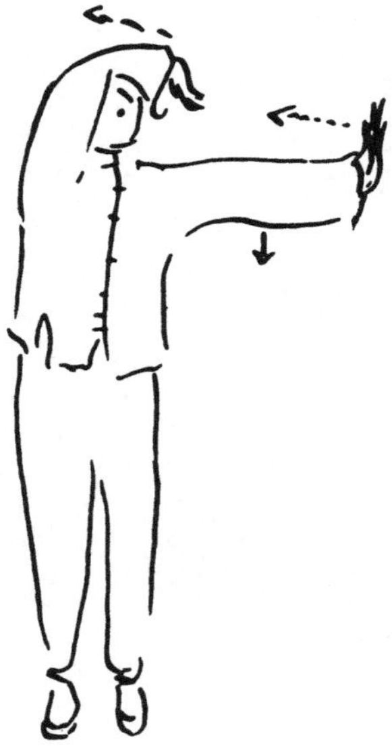

Figure 21

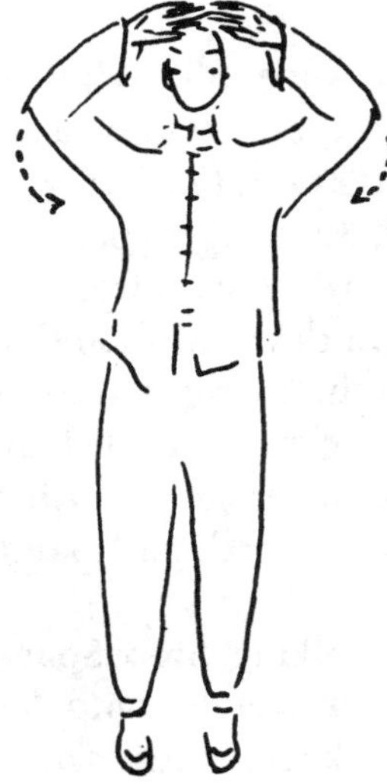

Figure 22

Figure 23

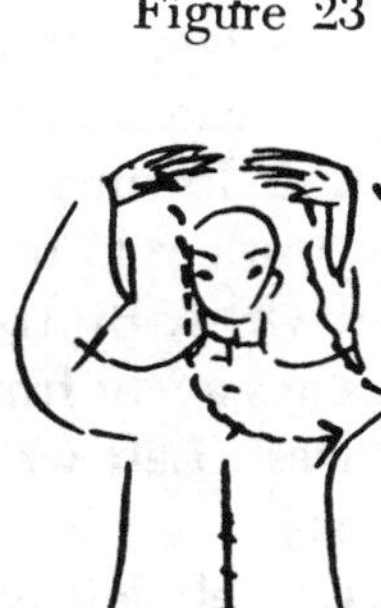

Turn torso to north. As you do this, bend left elbow and bring left hand to center of forehead, with palm north, so that fingers point to right finger tips. Finger tips do not touch each other; hands are a fist length away from forehead. The legs are straight. (Figure 22)

Bend both knees, keeping back straight. At the same time as you bend knees, move both hands: bend the wrists and turn hands so that palms face diagonally front-downward. At the same time as hands move, press elbows diagonally forward so that right elbow points northeast and left points northwest, both being at shoulder level. Make this movement with strength and hardness. Feel the hard contraction in muscles of upper arms. This contrasts with the light and soft movement you have been using up to now. Feel as if you were holding or pressing a huge ball between elbows and hands. Knees and hands move together. (Figure 23)

Form 8. Brush Knee Twist Step LOU HSI NIU PU

Right side

Keep weight on right leg with its bent knee. Shift right heel to east: this movement turns torso to face west, and at the same time, the weight is released from left leg. Then straighten left knee and flex foot. As body and legs turn to west, turn right palm inward toward forehead and turn left palm outward. Then circle left arm outward and downward and move right arm down to shoulder level. Continue the circle of left hand under right as right hand circles above left wrist. By this time you are facing west. Both hands are twelve inches away from chest. Right palm faces south with fingers pointing west. Left wrist is bent, with fingers north and palm west. (Figure 24)

Moving left leg west, place heel in Walking Step Space with straight knee and flexed foot. Then transfer weight onto left leg, bending left knee, and straightening right knee. Body slants on a diagonal toward west. As you step west both arms move: move right arm to west in line with right shoulder, turning palm to face west with fingers pointing upward. At the same time circle left arm with bent wrist downward, and place left hand in front of left thigh. Palm faces floor, with fingers pointing west. (Figure 25)

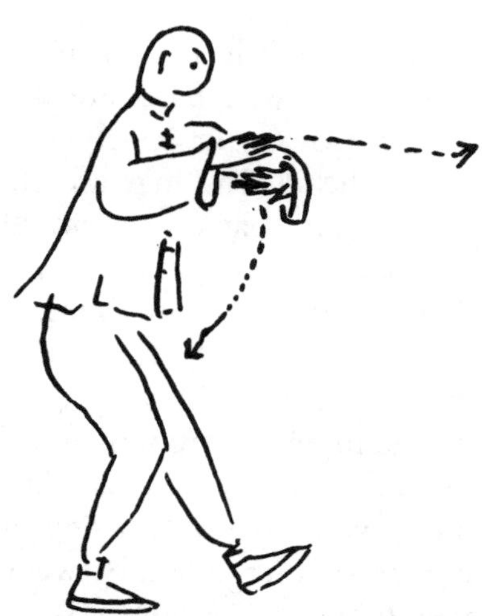

Figure 24

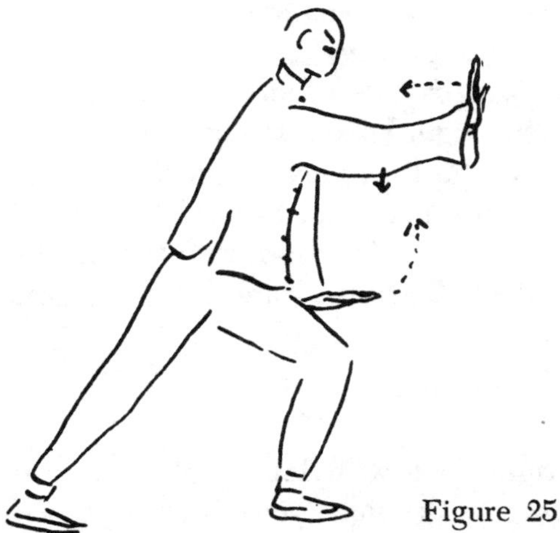

Figure 25

Form 9. Hand Strums the Lute SHOU HUI P'I-P'A

Shift weight back onto right leg, bending right knee, and at the same time, straighten left knee and flex foot. As legs move, both arms move: bring right arm inward twelve inches from face, keeping right palm facing west with fingers pointing up. Move left hand upward, and place finger tips at right pulse. Left palm faces inward toward the heart. Arms and legs move at the same time. (Figure 26)

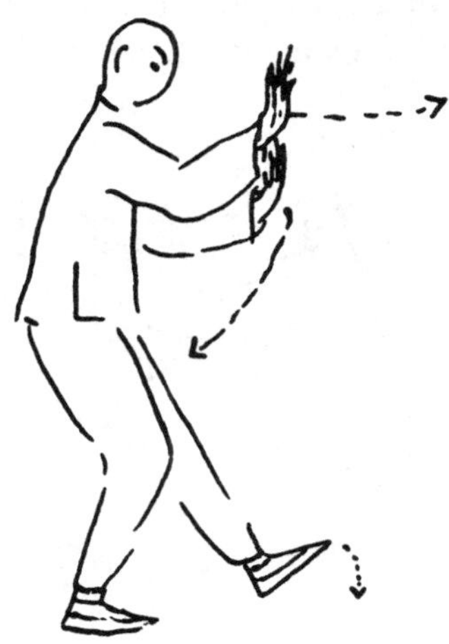

Figure 26

Form 10. Brush Knee Twist Step **LOU HSI NIU PU**

Same as Form 8, Figure 25

Transfer weight to left foot in the Walking Step (see page 29): left knee is bent, right knee is straight, and body slants on a diagonal forward. As you do this, move right arm west directly in line with right shoulder, turning palm to west with wrist shoulder high. At the same time, move left arm downward in front of left thigh with palm facing floor. Both arms and leg move and finish at the same time. (Figure 25)

Brush Knee Twist Step
On left side

Draw right foot with loose ankle in near left foot, without touching floor. At the same time both arms move: move left hand with fingers pointing west (palm is north) up to center, and move right hand (palm down) inward toward center, keeping wrist bent with fingers pointing south. Move left hand above right wrist. Both hands meet in center, twelve inches away from chest. (Figure 25–A)

(This position is opposite to that of Figure 25.) Move right leg forward west. Straightening knee and flexing foot, touch heel to floor in the Walking Step Space. Then transfer weight onto right foot, bending right knee and straightening left knee. Body slants forward on a diagonal. At the same time as legs move, both arms move: move left arm toward the west in line with left shoulder, turning palm to west, with wrist shoulder high; move right arm with bent wrist down in front of right thigh, palm facing floor with fingers pointing west. Both arms and legs move together.

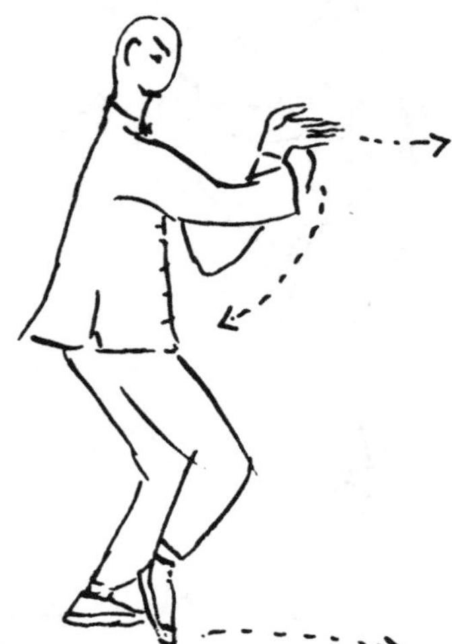

Figure 25A

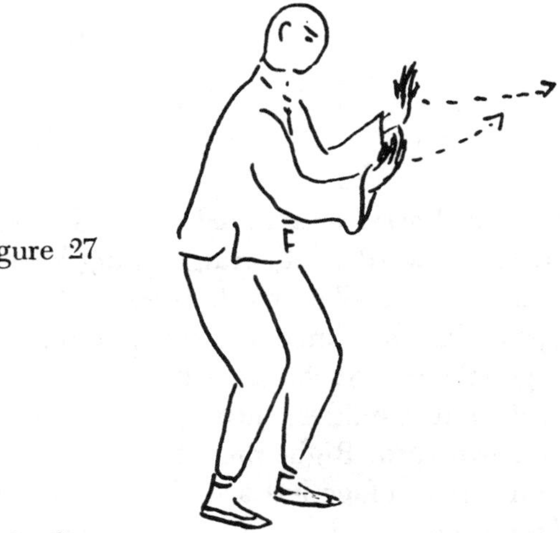

Figure 27

Brush Knee Twist Step
On right side

Draw left foot with loose ankle in toward right foot without touching floor. At the same time both arms move: move right hand up with fingers pointing west (palm is south) and move left hand inward toward the center of chest keeping wrist bent, fingers pointing north. Right hand moves above left wrist. Both hands meet in center, twelve inches away from chest. (This position is opposite to that of Figure 25–A)

Move left leg forward west. Straightening knee and flexing foot, touch heel to floor in the Walking Step Space. Then transfer weight onto left foot, bending left knee and straightening right knee. Body slants on a diagonal west. As you step west both arms move: move right arm west directly in line with right shoulder, turning palm to face west with wrist shoulder high, and move left arm downward in front of left thigh with palm facing floor, fingers pointing west. Both arms and legs move and finish at the same time. (Figure 25)

Form 11. Hand Strums the Lute SHOU HUI P'I-P'A

On left side

Keeping left knee bent, move the right foot and place it parallel and apart from left in your basic stance: both knees are bent and body is straight. Both arms move at the same time as right leg. Keeping palm west, move left arm up twelve inches from face, while you move right hand inward, turning palm inward, and place right finger tips near left pulse. Right palm faces heart. (Figure 27)

Form 12. Step Up, Parry, and Punch CHIN PU PAN LAN CH'UI

Move left leg forward west, straightening knee and flexing foot. Touch heel to floor in the Walking Step Space. Then transfer weight onto left foot, bending left knee and straightening right knee. Body slants on a diagonal west. At the same time, move both arms forward west in line with left shoulder; turn left palm to north with fingers pointing west-downward. Right fingers remain at left pulse: therefore, right palm turns to face left arm, south, and both elbows point downward. (Figure 28)

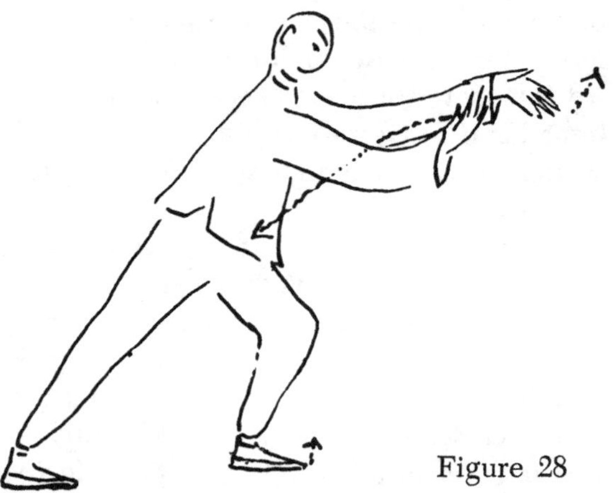

Figure 28

Shift weight back onto right leg, bending right knee, straightening left knee, and flexing left foot (Empty Step). At the same time, both arms move: draw right hand close along left forearm toward its elbow and then bring right hand down toward right hip, closing it gradually, so that when it reaches the hip the hand is a fist. Right elbow points to north; fist-palm is turned upward so that knuckles point to floor. While right arm moves, angle left hand so that fingers point west-upward. Do not move left arm out of its position. (Figure 29)

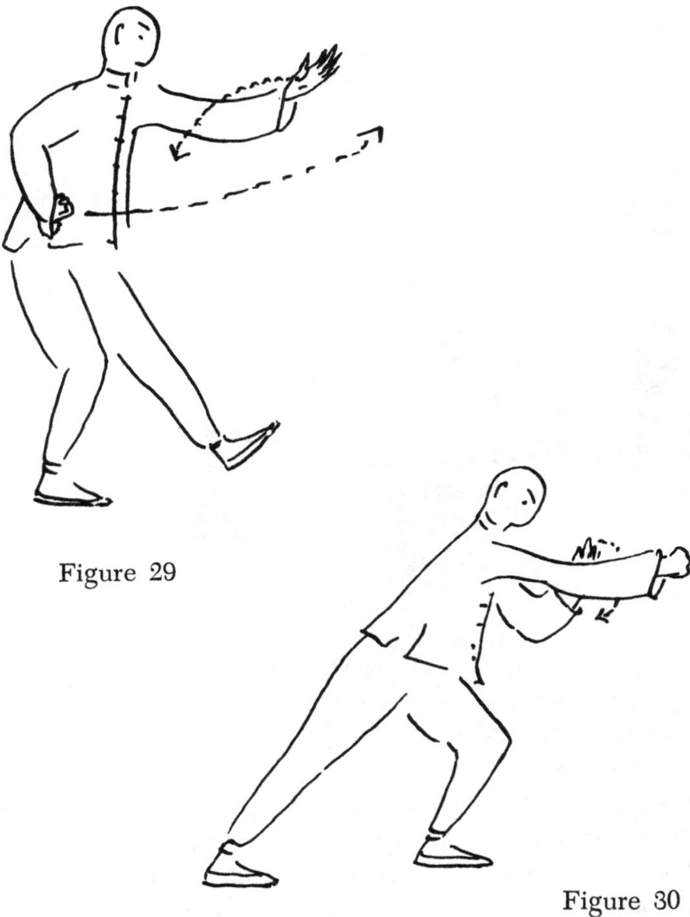

Figure 29

Figure 30

Shift weight forward onto left leg, bending left knee and straightening right knee. At the same time, both arms move: move right arm up west in line with right shoulder, with fist-palm facing south, elbow straight. Move left palm near inner side of right elbow; left wrist is bent with fingers pointing to ceiling. Arm movements and shifting of weight go together. (Figure 30)

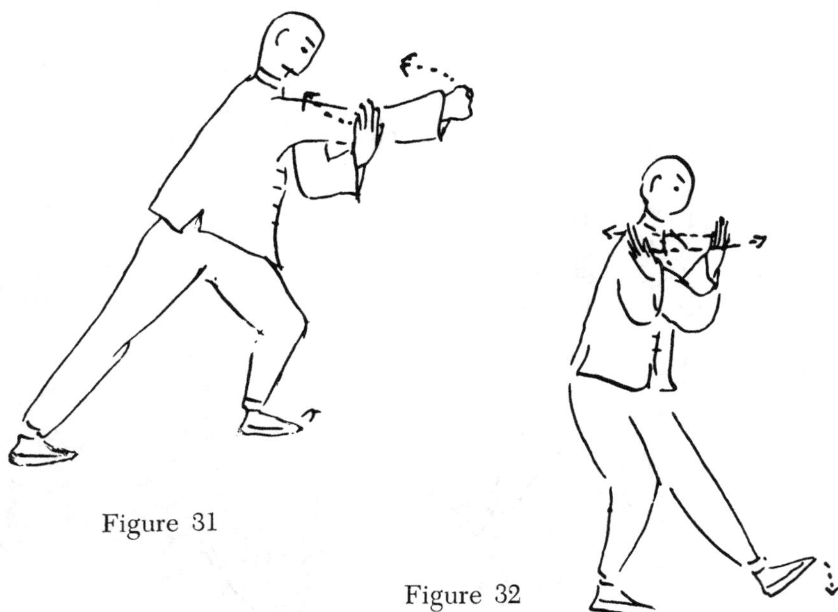

Figure 31

Figure 32

Form 13. As If You Were Shutting a Door JU FENG SZU PI

Do not move legs or torso. Move left hand under right arm to its outer side, and turn palm to face right elbow. (Figure 31)

Shift weight back onto right leg, bending right knee, and straighten left knee, flexing left foot. At the same time, both arms move: bend right elbow bringing the right fist in toward left shoulder, opening the fist gradually so that palm faces left shoulder, and move left palm, facing inward, in to face right shoulder. Left arm is on the outside of right arm. Both elbows are bent downward and forearms are crossed on a diagonal.

At the same time both arms move: move right hand in front of right shoulder with palm facing it and move left in front of left shoulder with palm facing it. Elbows are bent downward, wrists are straight, and fingers point to ceiling.

Then turn both palms to face west, keeping wrists straight and elbows down. All these arm movements are made as weight is shifted from left leg back to right leg with bent knee. (Figure 32)

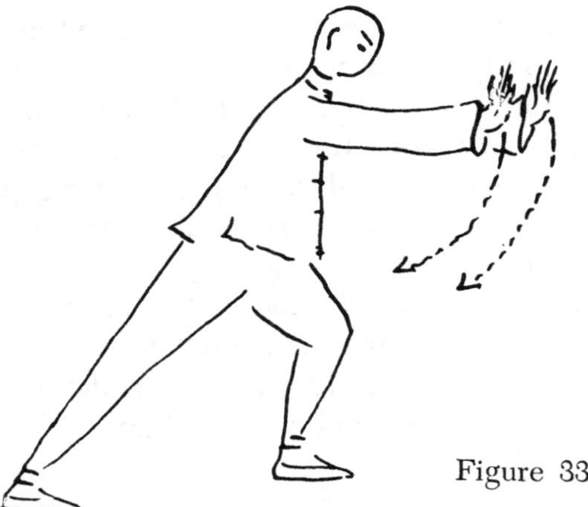

Figure 33

Form 14. Carry Tiger, Push Mountain PAO HU T'UI SHAN

Shift weight forward onto left leg, bending left knee and straightening right knee. At the same time, push both hands, which are facing west, forward shoulder high, to west, each arm in line with its shoulder: wrists are shoulder high, and body slants forward on a diagonal west. (Figure 33)

Keep weight on left leg. Bend torso down, moving arms at same time, and lower arms so that palms face floor at knee level. Arms are perpendicular to floor. (Figure 34)

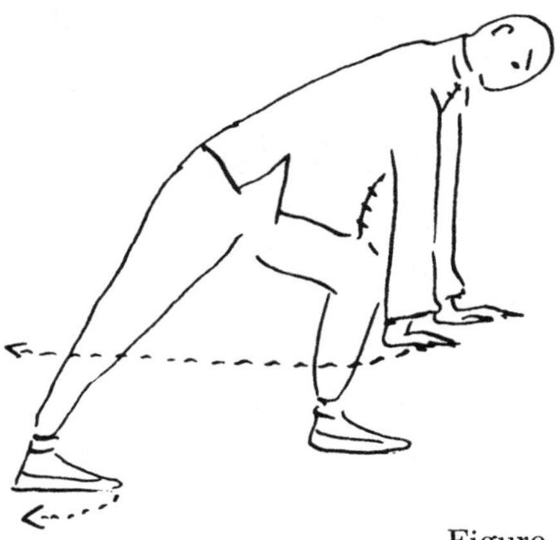

Figure 34

Form 15. Cross Hands **SHIH TZU SHOU**

Turn right toes to north and at the same time shift weight onto right leg, bending right knee and straightening left knee. With these movements, torso moves to north, still remaining bent over; do not lower head. At the same time as torso and right toes move, move right hand to right side of right leg, keeping palm down. Right fingers now point east. Left hand remains at left side; palm is down with fingers pointing west. (Figure 35)

Turn left toes to north, and at the same time, gradually raise the torso to an upright position, bringing arms up sideways, shoulder high. Then move them forward north, shoulder high. Straighten wrists as you raise torso and arms. (Figure 36)

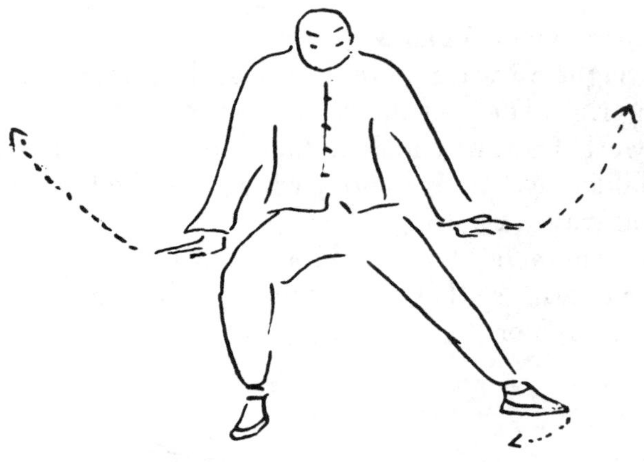

Figure 35

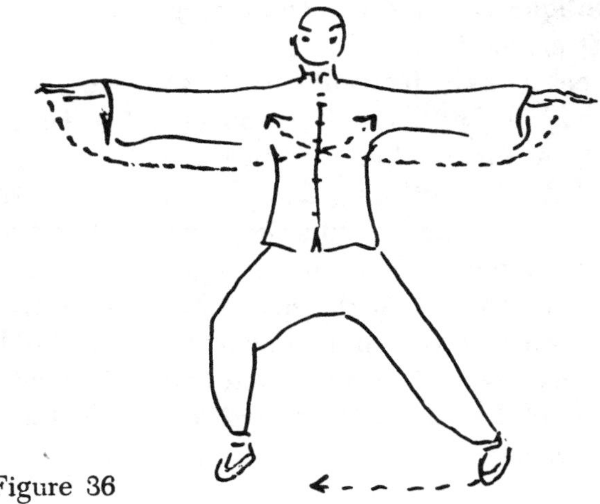

Figure 36

Keeping right knee bent, place left foot parallel to right and apart from it in your basic stance. Both knees are bent. At the same time, bring both arms inward, crossing forearms diagonally: right forearm is on the outside of left forearm, left palm faces east on a slant, and right palm faces west on a slant. The V cross of the arms is just below chin level about twelve inches away: elbows are high and back is straight. (Figure 37)

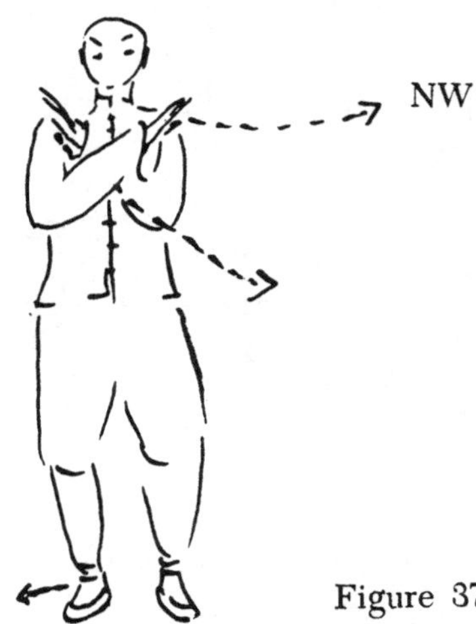

Figure 37

Form 16. Oblique Brush Knee Twist Step HSIEH LOU HSI NIU PU
To northwest on right side

Move heel of right foot outward to southeast, keeping weight on right leg with its bent knee. This movement releases weight from left leg and turns torso to face northwest.

Move left leg to northwest, straightening knee and flexing foot. Place heel on floor in the Walking Step Space. Then transfer weight onto left foot, bending knee and straightening right knee. Body slants forward northwest. At the same time, both arms move: move right arm forward northwest in line with right shoulder, turning palm to face northwest, and move left arm with bent wrist downward in front of left thigh; fingers point northwest and palm is down. (Figure 38)

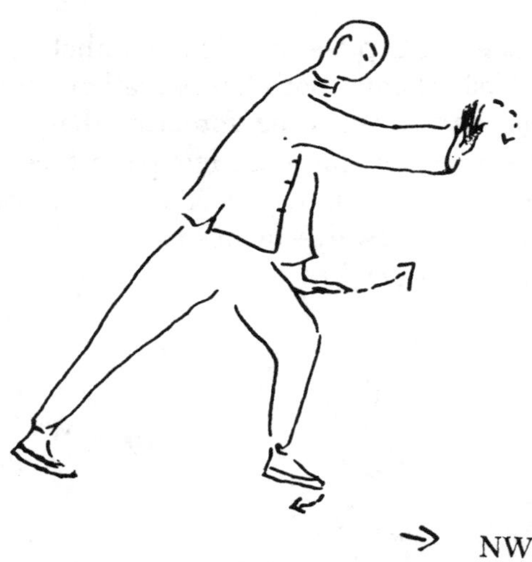

Figure 38

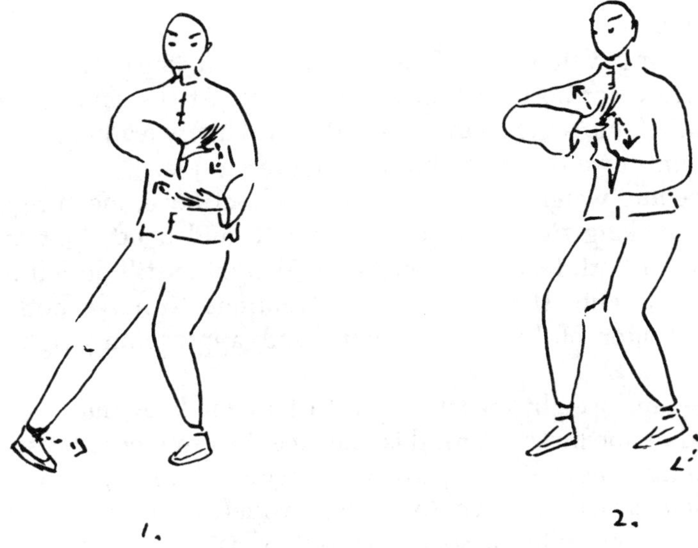

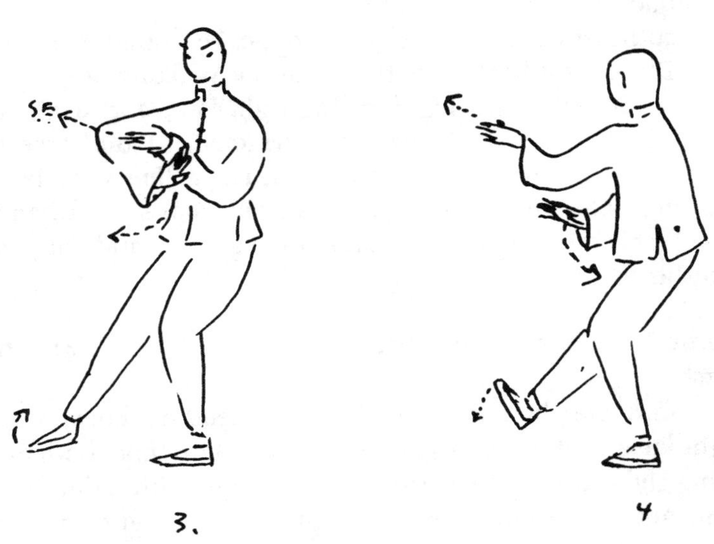

Figure 39

Toe—Heel—Heel—Step
(See page 31.)

Keeping weight on left leg with its bent knee, move left toes inward to point northeast. Straighten torso. At the same time, both arms move: move left hand upward with fingers leading, and move right hand inward toward body. (Figure 39–1)

Keeping weight on left leg with its bent knee, move right heel inward, making right foot parallel to left, and bend right knee, so that toes of both feet point northeast. Weight is still on left leg and torso is straight. At the same time, continue to move both hands toward center of body, with left hand approaching right wrist. (Figure 39–2)

Keeping weight on left leg with its bent knee, move left heel outward to northwest. With this movement torso faces east and right knee straightens. Feet are now in T position (see page 29). At the same time, arms move: continue to move left hand over right wrist, with left fingers pointing southeast; right wrist is bent. (Figure 39–3)

Weight is still on left leg with its bent knee. Turning torso to face southeast, raise right toes off floor. At the same time, both arms move: move right arm with bent wrist down toward front of right thigh, and move left arm up toward southeast. (Figure 39–4)

Oblique Brush Knee Twist Step
To southeast on left side, position opposite to that of Figure 38

Place right heel to southeast, in the Walking Step Space. Transfer weight onto right leg, bending right knee and straightening left knee. Body slants southeast on a diagonal. At the same time, both arms move: move left arm to southeast in line with left shoulder, turning palm out to face southeast; and move right hand down to front of right thigh, with palm facing floor and fingers pointing southeast.

Form 17. Grasping the Bird's Tail LAN CH'ÜEH WEI
First

Shift weight back onto left leg, bending knee, straightening right knee, and flexing right foot. At the same time, both arms move: bring right arm up to southeast, chin high, with palm facing northeast, and place left fingers at right pulse. (Figure 7—except that here you face the southeast diagonal instead of east.)

Keep the relationship of hands the same. Bending both elbows downward and slightly out, draw both arms inward toward body at chin level. Do not come too close to your face.

Turn right palm up and left palm down. As hands move, angle left hand so that it is at right angles to right wrist; therefore, left elbow points northeast. (Figure 8, except that here you face southeast.)

Grasping the Bird's Tail
Second

Transfer weight onto the right leg, bending right knee and straightening left knee, with body on a slant diagonally toward southeast. As the same time as you do this, stretch right arm to the east, chin high, straightening elbow. Keep left fingers above right pulse. (Figure 9, except that here you face east.)

Move both arms in a horizontal circle, chin high, from east to southeast, to south, to west. When arms reach south, bend right elbow downward and bend right wrist so that palm faces upward. Both right and left fingers point west at end of horizontal circling. Left arm is adjusted to movement of right arm, because left fingers always remain near right pulse.

As you make circling movement from south to west, shift weight back onto left leg, bending left knee, and straighten right knee, flexing foot. (Figure 10, except that here you face southeast.)

Grasping the Bird's Tail
Third

Pivot on right heel, turning toes to east, and place foot on floor. At the same time, raise right arm with palm leading up toward ceiling; circle it up, over, and down toward the east, straightening arm as you do so. Stop at a place where right wrist is slightly above shoulder height. (Figure 11, except that here you face toward east.)

As you are approaching this last position, bend right knee, placing weight on right leg; and at the same time bend right wrist and lower right hand downward so that fingers point downward. As hand bends down, place all fingers close together over thumb as if grasping it. Right arm remains in its position when wrist bends and fingers move. Left fingers are still at right pulse, with palm toward the face. Left wrist is straight and arm is curved. (Figure 11)

Form 18. The Single Whip **TAN PIEN**

Holding weight on right leg, draw left foot close to right—without touching floor. Continue to move left leg: place it in northwest diagonal in the Walking Step Space. Straighten left knee and place foot parallel to right foot. Body is on a diagonal slant toward the east. While moving left leg, move left arm in a downward curve, in toward the body, waist high. Continue to move it, raising arm upward toward the north. Arm is curved, palm faces upward toward the face. (Figure 12, except that here the direction is east.)

Pivoting on left heel, turn toes toward north, at the same time, bending left knee to equal bend of right knee. Weight is equal on both legs. Feet are separated by a distance equal to twice the length of the foot. Back is straight. As you move left foot, turn left hand to face palm north. Now both arms are on the same level; wrists are slightly higher than shoulder level. Right arm is toward east in grasping position, and left palm faces north. Right toes point east, and left toes point north. Body is turned to northeast. (Figure 40)

Movements of Head and Eyes for Form 18

Look at left palm; keep eyes on it as arm moves to north. Turn head from right to left sides, but do *not* bend it downward when eyes look downward. The top of head is kept level as head turns. When left palm faces north eyes will then look at back of hand. (Figures 12 and 13, except that here the direction is north.) Eyes, head, arm, legs and body movements must be synchronized.

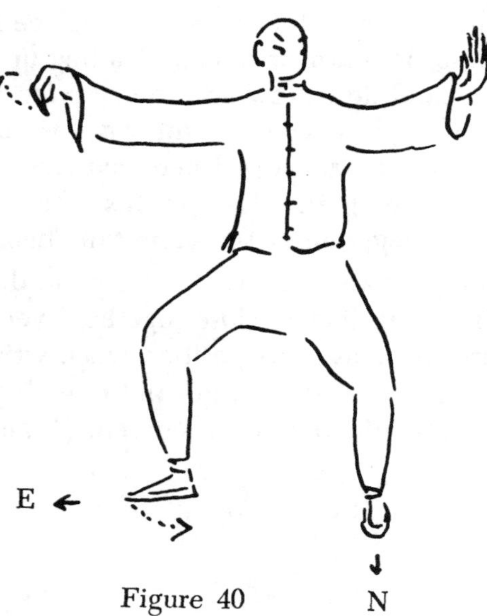

Figure 40

SERIES II

Form 19. Fist Under Elbow — CHOU TI K'AN CH'UI

Move right toes to point north; at the same time shift weight to left leg, bending left knee a bit more, and straighten right knee. This movement turns torso to face north. As you shift weight, open right hand so that palm faces upward and right wrist is straight. Foot, weight, torso, and hand move together. (Figure 41)

Move left toes to point west, keeping left knee bent with weight remaining on left. This movement turns torso (which is on a diagonal) to face west. At the same time as toes and torso move, turn left palm upward with straightened wrist and move both arms with torso. Keep arms outstretched at shoulder level as torso faces toward west: left arm extends to south, right arm extends to north, and both palms face up. (Figure 42)

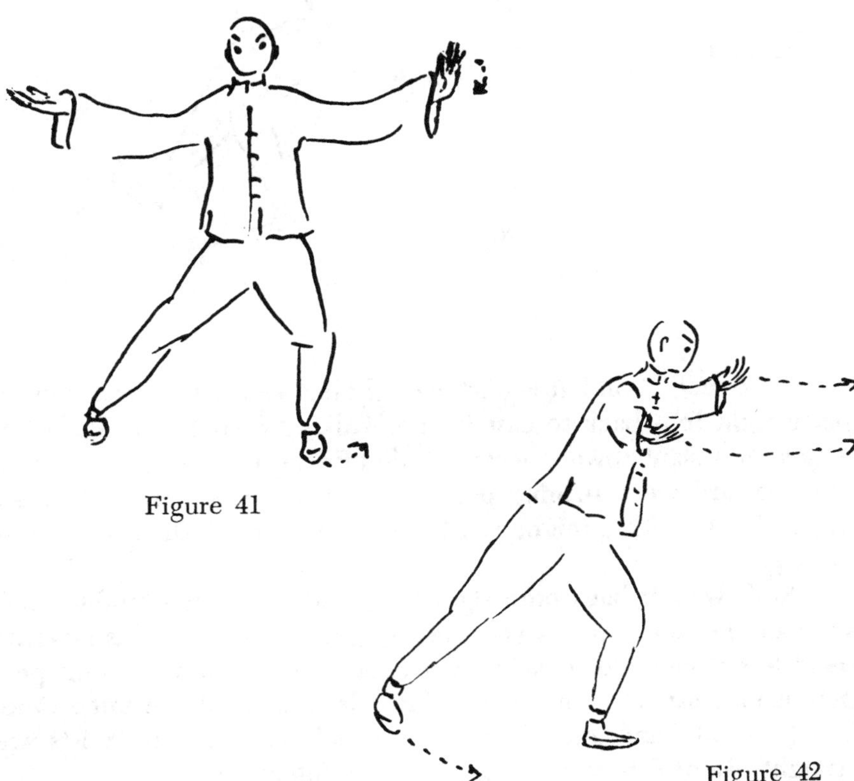

Figure 41

Figure 42

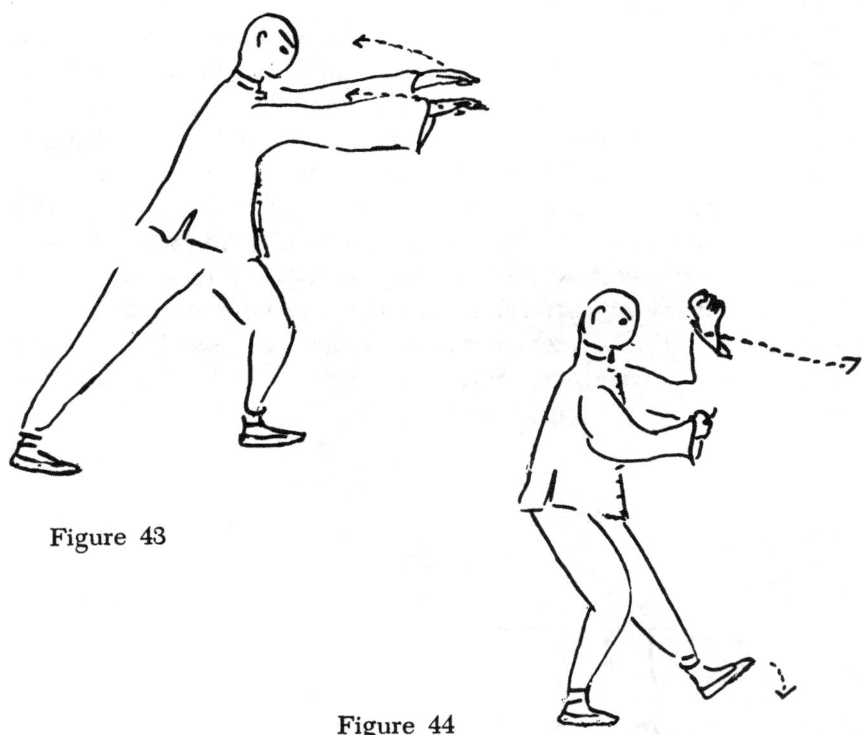

Figure 43

Figure 44

Hold weight on left leg. Move right leg, and straightening knee, place right foot back to east in the Walking Step Space. Body remains on a slant toward west. While moving right leg, move both arms toward west, turning palms downward. Keep arms shoulder high. Hands with straight wrists are shoulder width apart. (Figure 43)

Shift weight back onto right leg, bending knee; straighten left knee and flex left foot. As you shift weight, draw both arms inward: bend left elbow and make a right angle with forearm up in a perpendicular; fist the hand, facing fist-palm north. At the same time, fist the right hand and place it under left elbow; both wrists are straight. Right fist–palm faces inward. (Figure 44)

Form 20. Brush Knee Twist Step LOU HSI NIU PU

Going backward on left side

Shift weight forward onto left foot, bending left knee, and straighten right knee; body is on a slant forward west in the Walking Step position. At the same time, move left arm to west shoulder high, straightening elbow and opening left hand: palm faces north with fingers to west. Right fist remains under left elbow. (Figure 45)

Draw left arm slightly inward toward shoulder by bending elbow downward, and bend wrist so that fingers remain pointing to west. Wrist is shoulder high; right fist is still under left elbow. At the same time shift weight back onto right leg, bending knee, and straighten left knee, flexing foot. (Figure 46)

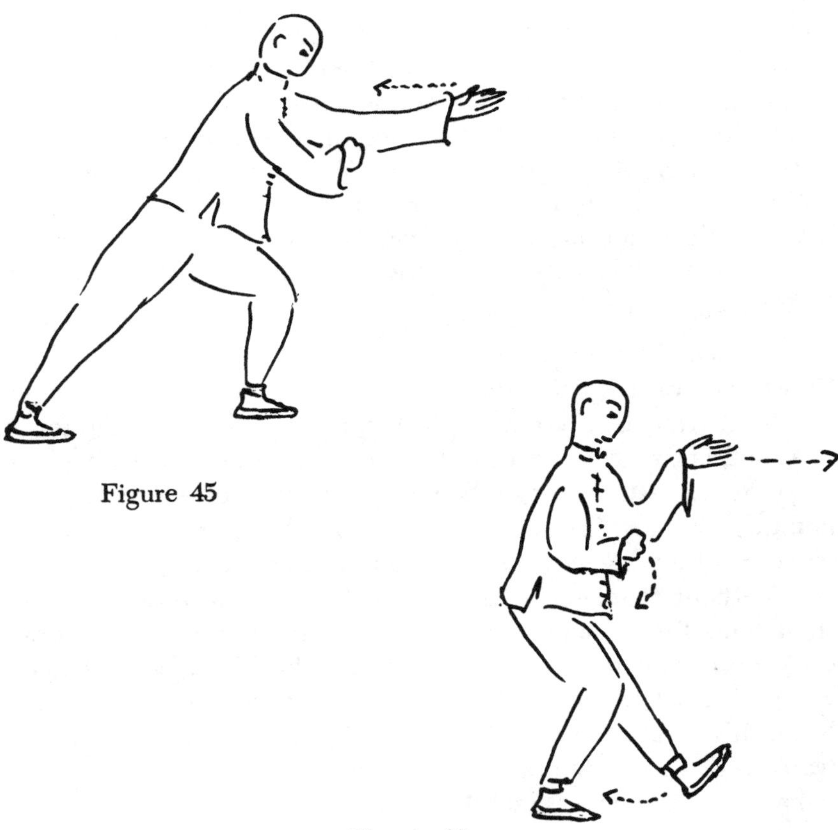

Figure 45

Figure 46

Without touching floor, draw left foot with loose ankle close to right foot. At the same time continue to draw left arm inward toward left shoulder; open right hand gradually and start to move it downward toward right thigh. (Figure 47)

Weight remains on right leg with its bent knee. Place left foot backward behind body, to east, in the Walking Step Space, and straighten knee. Body slants forward west. As the left leg moves, move left arm forward west in line with left shoulder, turning hand to face west, while right hand finishes its movement at front of right thigh, with palm down and fingers west. (Figure 48)

Brush Knee Twist Step
Going backward on right side

Shift weight back onto left leg, bending left knee; straighten right knee and flex right foot. Draw left hand inward to center, twelve inches from chest, keeping elbow high; palm faces west with fingers pointing north. At the same time, move right hand upward above left wrist, pointing fingers west, with palm south. (Figure 49)

Without touching floor, draw right foot with loose angle close to left. Keep weight on left leg. Place right foot behind toward east in the Walking Step Space, straightening knee. At the same time, both arms continue to move: move right arm forward in line with right shoulder, turning palm to west. Circle left arm downward to front of left thigh, with palm down and fingers pointing to west. (Figure 25)

Brush Knee Twist Step
Going backward on left side

Shift weight back onto right leg, bending knee; straighten left knee and flex foot. Draw right hand inward to center, twelve inches away from chest, keeping elbow high: palm faces west with fingers pointing south. At the same time, move left hand upward above right wrist, pointing fingers west, with palm facing north.

Without touching floor, draw left foot with loose ankle in to right foot. Keep weight on right leg. Place left foot back toward east in the Walking Step Space, straightening knee. Body slants forward west. At the same time, both arms continue to move: move left arm forward west in line with left shoulder, turning palm toward west. Circle right arm downward to front of right thigh, with palm down, and fingers pointing west. (Figure 48)

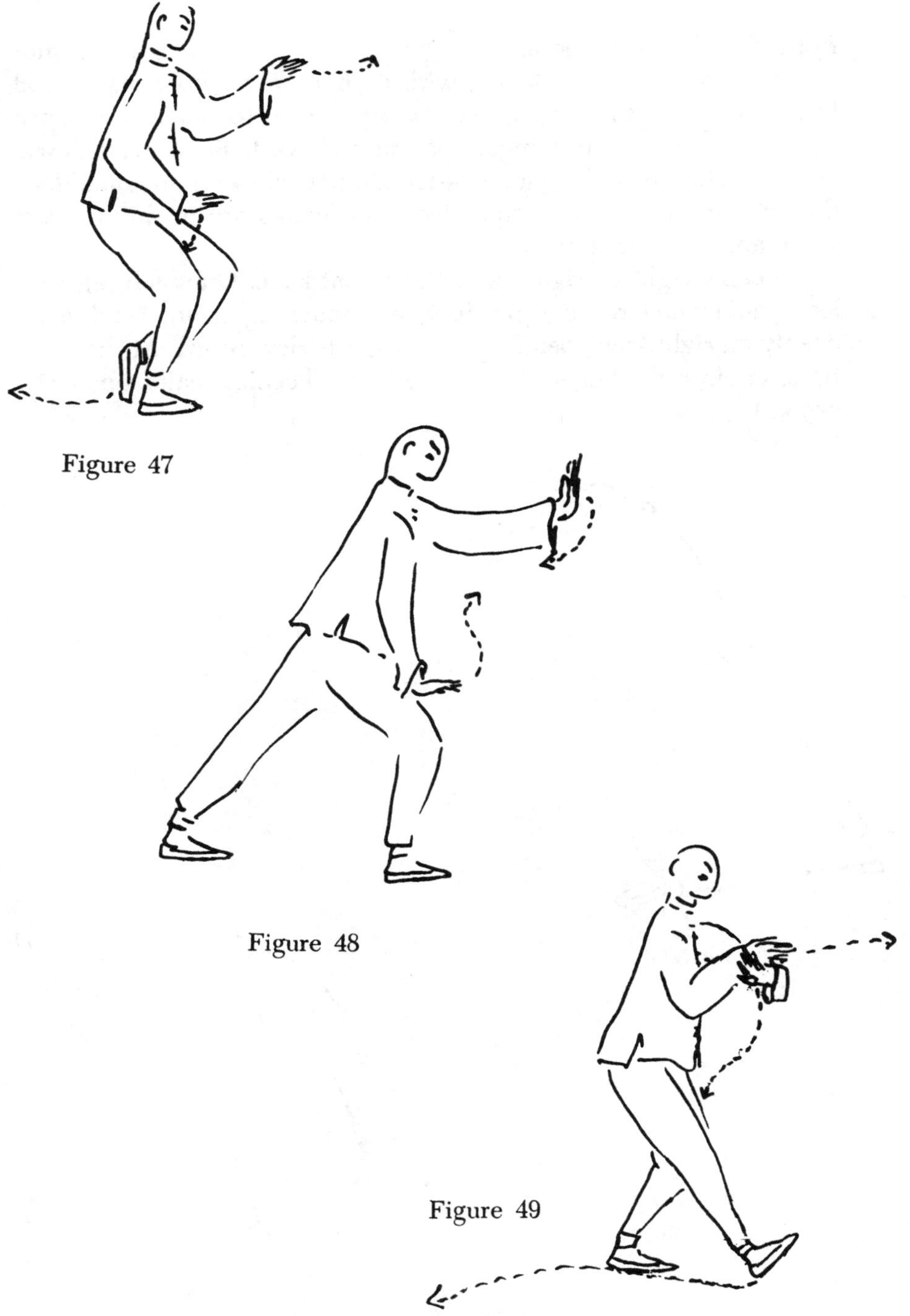

Figure 47

Figure 48

Figure 49

Form 21. Flying Oblique HSIEH FEI SHIH

Keep weight on right leg with its bent knee. Foot, hand, and head move together. Turn toes of right foot to northwest. Turn right palm up, keeping fingers pointing to west. Bend head down, and turn chin toward right shoulder. Do not move arm or shoulders; do not shift weight from right leg. Movements are made in ankle, wrist, and neck. (Figure 50)

Keep weight on right leg with its bent knee. Draw left leg with loose ankle inward to right foot, not touching floor. Bend more deeply on right knee, bending torso slightly downward. At the same time, circle right fingers inward to body, keeping palm up. (Figure 51)

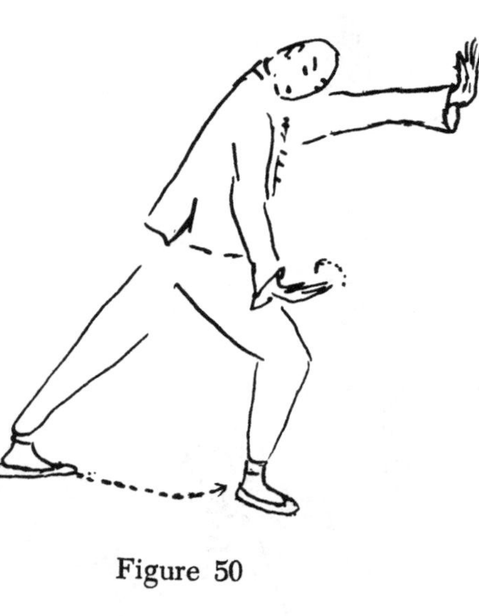

Figure 50

Figure 51

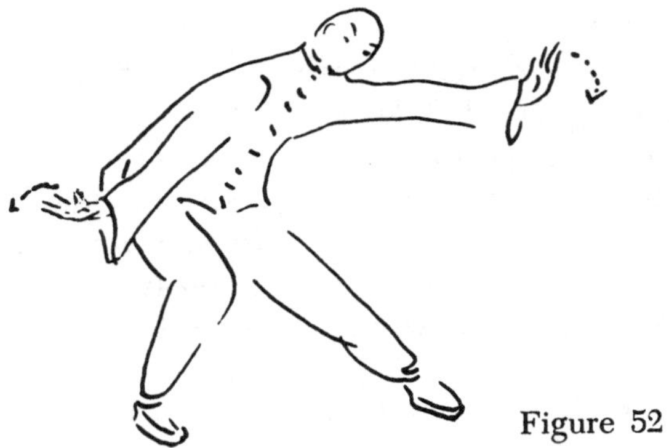

Figure 52

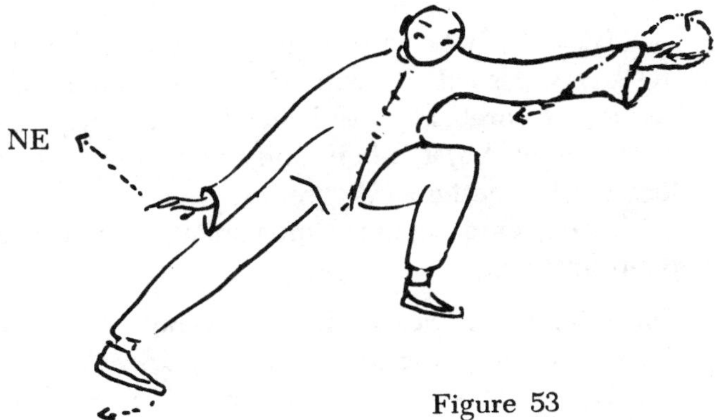

Figure 53

Move left leg outward toward southwest, as far as it can go with a straight knee. Place left foot parallel to right foot. Now both feet point northwest. At the same time continue to circle right hand with palm up inward to northeast; fingers point to northeast. (Figure 52)

Shift weight onto left leg, bending left knee and straightening right knee. Bend torso forward and sit as low as you can on left leg: body faces northwest. Head looks northeast. At the same time, as body lowers over onto left side, turn left palm up with fingers pointing west, and straighten wrist. At the same time, turn right palm down, with fingers pointing northeast. Right arm is parallel to right leg. Look at back of right hand. All these movements finish together. (Figure 53)

Form 22. Raise Hands and Step Up T'I SHOU SHANG SHIH
The same as Form 6, Figures 16, 17, 18

Turn right toes to point north and shift weight onto right leg, bending right knee, and straighten left knee. On this movement, keep body low; turn torso to face north. Then turn toes of left foot to point north. At the same time as legs move, both arms move: bring right arm forward in a curve, shoulder high, fifteen inches from body. Move left hand with palm turned toward northeast, toward inner curve of right elbow. Left elbow points downward and right elbow is shoulder high. (Figure 16)

Draw left foot up and place it parallel and apart from right foot, in the basic stance. Both knees are bent equally and torso is curved forward north. At the same time, the arms complete the movements described above: right arm is curved forward shoulder high, and left palm is at inner curve of right elbow. (Figure 17)

Raise body to an upright position, at the same time straightening knees. Also at the same time, lift curved right arm to a position just above forehead, and lower left arm, with palm down, to front of left thigh: wrist is bent and fingers point north. Arms, body, and legs finish together. (Figure 18)

Then, as a separate movement, turn the right hand to face palm upward.

Form 23. White Stork Flaps Its Wings PAI HAO LIANG CH'IH
Same as Form 7, Figures 19, 20, 21, 22, 23

Do not move right arm from its place above forehead for the next sequences.

Bend torso forward down, and, at the same time, move left arm away from thigh so that it is perpendicular to floor, palm facing floor. (Figure 19)

Keep arms in same relative positions. Twist torso around to west, keeping body low. Arms move with body. Now left fingers point west. (Figure 20)

Lift torso up erect, remaining turned west. At the same time bring straight left arm up shoulder high. Left wrist is bent with palm west, and fingers point upward. (Figure 21)

Turn torso to north. As you do this, bend left elbow and bring left hand to center of forehead, with palm north, so that left fingers point to right fingers. Finger tips of hands are close but do not touch. Hands are a fist length away from forehead. (Figure 22)

Bend both knees, keeping back straight. At the same time, move both hands: bend wrists and turn hands so that palms face diagonally front-downward. At the same time as hands move, press elbows diagonally forward so that right elbow points northeast and left points northwest, both being at shoulder level. Make this movement with strength and hardness. Feel the contraction in the muscles of upper arms. This contrasts with the light and soft movement you have been using up to now. Feel as if you were holding or pressing a huge ball between elbows and hands. Knees and hands move together. (Figure 23)

Form 24. Brush Knee Twist Step LOU HSI NIU PU

Right side—same as in Form 8, Figures 24, 25

Keep weight on right with its bent knee. Shift right heel to the east. This movement turns torso to face west, and at the same time, the weight is released from left leg. Then straighten left knee and flex foot. As body and legs turn to west, turn right palm inward toward forehead, and turn left palm outward. Then circle left arm outward and downward, and move right arm down to shoulder level. Continue the circle of left hand under the right hand as right hand circles above left wrist. By this time you are facing west. Both hands are twelve inches away from chest: right palm faces south with fingers pointing west. Left wrist is bent, with fingers north and palm west. (Figure 24)

Moving left leg west, place heel in the Walking Step Space, with straight knee and flexed foot. Then transfer weight onto left leg, bending left knee, and straightening right knee. Body slants forward west. As you step west, both arms move: move right arm to west in line with right shoulder, turning palm to face west with fingers pointing upward. At the same time, circle left arm with bent wrist downward, and place left hand in front of left thigh. Palm faces floor with fingers pointing west. (Figure 25)

Form 25. Hand Strums the Lute SHOU HUI P'I-P'A

Same as Form 9, Figure 26

Shift weight back onto right leg, bending right knee, and at the same time, straighten left knee and flex foot. As legs move, both arms move: bring right arm inward twelve inches from face, keeping right palm facing west with fingers pointing up. Move left hand upward, and place finger tips at right pulse; left palm faces inward toward heart. Arms and legs move at the same time. (Figure 26)

Form 26. Needle at the Bottom of the Sea **HAI TI CHEN**

Draw left foot with loose ankle close to right foot, touching toes lightly on floor. Weight is on right leg. At the same time, lower torso by bending right knee more deeply, and lean torso forward on a diagonal. Keep spine straight—do not curve the back. On body and leg movement, move both arms: turning right palm south and left palm north, move right arm diagonally downward, with straight wrist, and gradually straighten right elbow. At the same time, move left palm close along right forearm to right inner elbow: left wrist bends gradually. Right arm is straight; left wrist and elbow are bent. Arms, leg, and body finish together. (Figure 54)

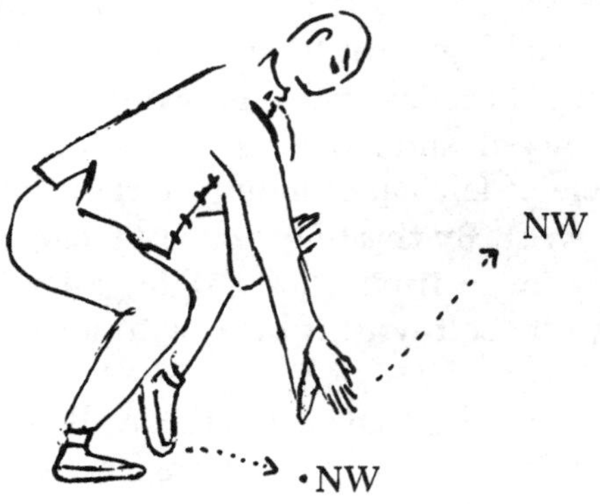

Figure 54

Form 27. Fan Through the Back **SHAN T'UNG PEI**

Keep weight on right leg. Raise torso and direct it to northwest angle. At same time, lift up both arms, pointing right fingers to northwest angle, at shoulder level; as right fingers point northwest left hand remains at right inner elbow.

Then place left foot in front of right, with left heel in line with right toes, turning left toes inward to point northwest. Straighten left knee. Right knee is close to left leg. Head looks northwest. (Figure 55)

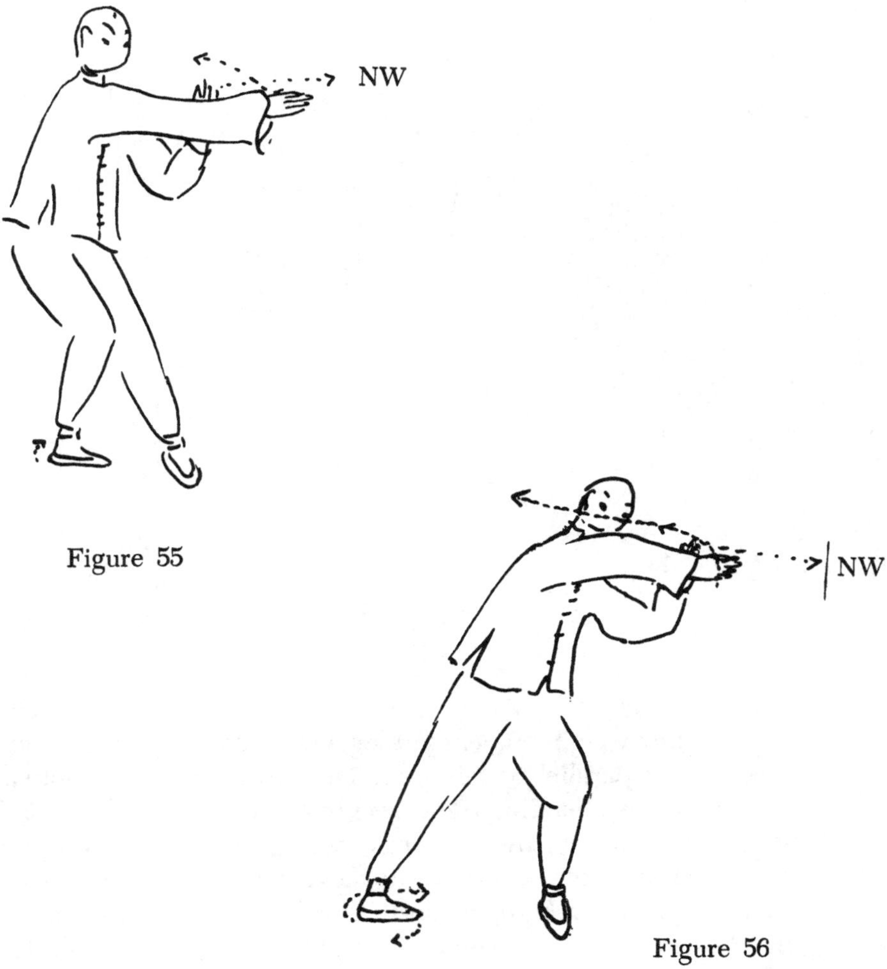

Figure 55

Figure 56

Shift weight onto left leg, bending left knee and straightening right knee. At the same time, begin to move both arms: slide (do not touch) left fingers along right forearm toward northwest and draw right arm to right side. Left finger tips are at right palm when left knee is bent and right knee is straight. (Figure 56)

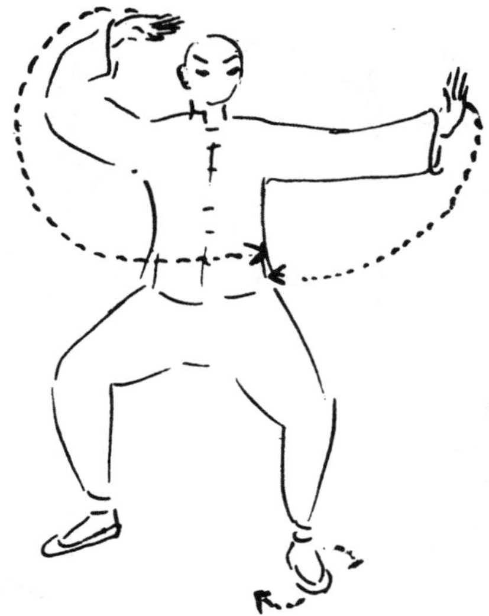

Figure 57

Keeping weight on bent left leg, move right heel slightly inward, making foot parallel to left foot. Then turn right toes outward to point northeast, bending right knee to equal left knee bend. You are now seated evenly on both legs, facing northeast. As you move right heel and toes, continue to move both arms: move left arm, which is shoulder high, to northwest with palm facing northwest and fingers up, and move curved right arm forehead high, to right side of head; then turn right palm outward and up, when arm gets into its position. Left arm is straight, and right arm is curved. Eyes look at back of left hand. (Figure 57)

Form 28. Turn Body—Throw Fist FAN SHEN P'IEH SHEN CH'UI

Keeping weight on left leg with bent knee, move left toes inward to northeast; then move left heel outward to west, and on this heel movement straighten right knee. Keep right foot on floor. As left toes and heel move, upper torso is shifted to face northeast; head remains looking north. While you move left toes and heel, both arms move: circle left arm downward; make hand into a fist and place it near left hip bone, with fist-palm facing down. Circle right arm, making hand into a fist, outward to east, then downward and inward toward left hip. Place right fist above left, with fist-palm down. Both fists arrive in position at the same time, with movements of left toes and heel. When fists meet, pull shoulders forward, moving elbows slightly forward. Use a hard force, similar to "pressing the ball," as in Form 7. (Figure 58)

Move right toes to point east, shifting weight onto right leg, bending right knee, and straightening left knee. Body slants forward east. At the same time, both arms move: move right fist up to east, chin high, with fist-palm facing east; wrist is bent. Move left fist, gradually opening hand and spreading fingers wide apart. Place it behind right fist: wrist is bent; left palm is behind right fist, with left fingers pointing upward. Both elbows are low. (Figure 59)

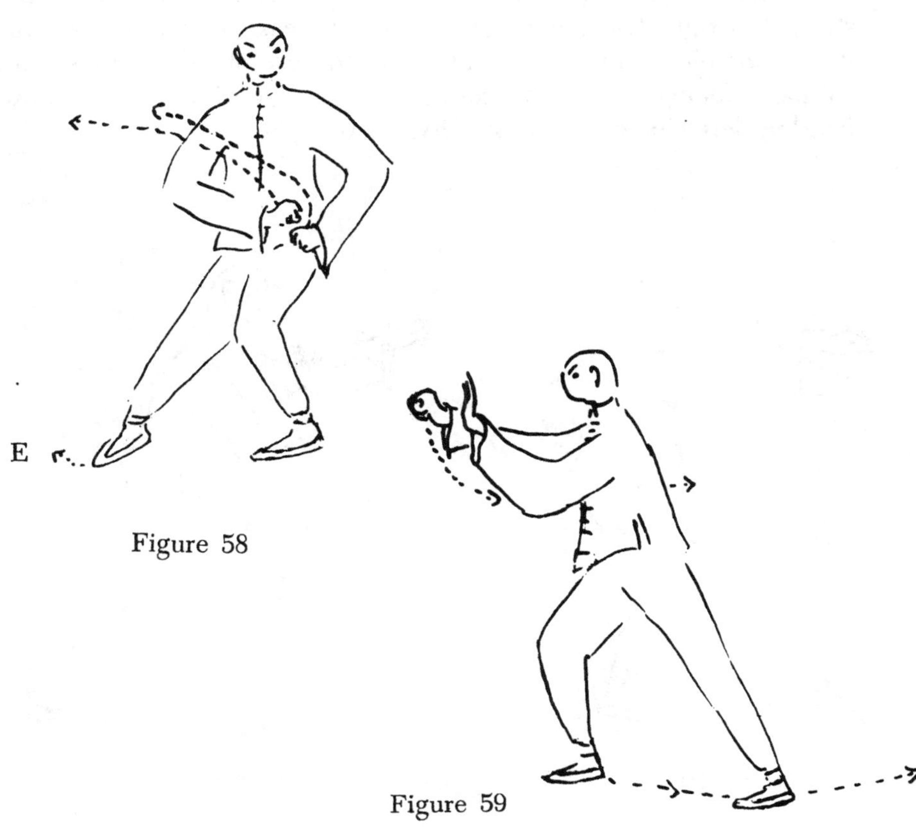

Figure 58

Figure 59

Form 29. Step Up, Parry, and Punch CHIN PU PAN LAN CH'UI

Shift weight back onto left leg, bending knee, straightening right leg, and flexing foot. At the same time, both hands move: turn left palm to face south and gradually place fingers together; turn right fist to face left palm. Draw right fist along left forearm (not touching it) and start to draw it back toward right hip, turning fist-palm upward, elbow moving back to point west. At the same time, as right arm is drawing back, draw right foot with loose ankle back to left foot (not touching floor).

Do not move left arm. Step right foot backward in Walking Step Space; place weight on right leg, bending right knee, straightening left knee, and flexing foot. On this last shifting of weight onto right leg, draw right fist to right hip, with elbow back to point west. Fist-palm faces upward; left arm remains forward east, in line with left shoulder. (Figure 60)

Shift weight forward onto left leg, bending its knee, and straighten right knee. Body slants forward east. At the same time, both arms move: bring right fist forward east, shoulder high, with fist-palm facing north, and move left palm to right inner elbow, bending left elbow and wrist. (Figure 61)

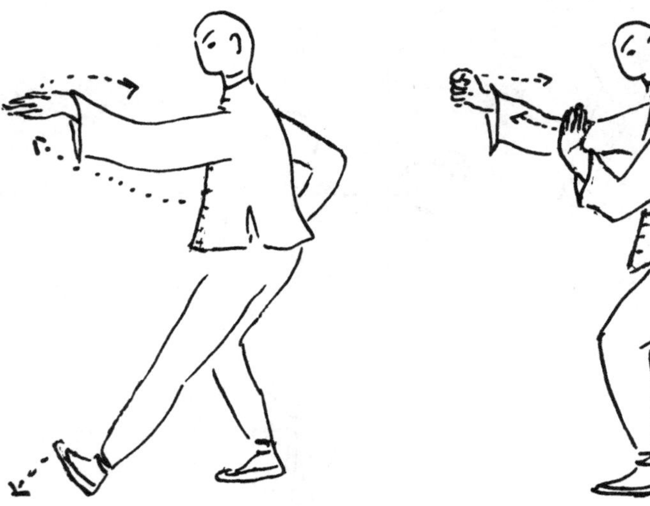

Figure 60

Figure 61

Form 30. Grasping the Bird's Tail LAN CH'ÜEH WEI

Same as Forms 2, 3, 4, Figures 7, 8, 9, 10

Shift weight back onto right leg, bending right knee, straightening left knee, and flexing foot. At the same time, move left fingers to right pulse and open right hand with fingers pointing east.

Keep the relationship of hands the same: move both arms inward toward the body at chin level, with both elbows bent downward and slightly out. Do not come too close to body. (Figure 7)

Turn right palm up and left palm down. As you move hands, angle left hand so that it is at right angles to right wrist and left elbow points north. At the same time as hands turn, shift weight forward onto left leg, bending left knee and straightening right knee; body is on a diagonal forward to east. Then draw right foot with loose ankle close to left foot. (Figure 8 for arms only)

Place right heel forward east in the Walking Step Space, bending right knee and straightening left knee. Body slants forward. At the same time as you step forward, stretch right arm to northeast, straightening right elbow. Keep left fingers at right wrist. (Figure 9)

Circle both arms horizontally, chin high, going from northeast to east, to south, to southwest. When arms reach south, bend right elbow downward, bending right wrist so that palm faces upward. Left fingers stay at right pulse. Left arm is adjusted to movement of right arm. (Figure 10)

As you are circling, when arms move from south to southwest, shift weight back onto left leg, bending left knee, and straighten right knee, flexing foot. (Figure 10)

Pivoting on right heel, turn right toes to northeast and place foot on floor. At the same time, raise right arm, with palm leading, up toward ceiling. Circle it over and down toward northeast, straightening arm as you do so, and stop in position when right wrist is slightly above shoulder height. (Figure 11)

As you are approaching this last position with right arm, bend right knee, placing weight on right leg, and straighten left knee. At the same time, bend right wrist and lower hand, making fingers point downward, and place all fingers over thumb in Grasping position: right arm remains in place while hand moves. Left fingers remain near right pulse; left palm faces your face. Left wrist is straight; arm is curved. (Figure 11)

Form 31. The Single Whip **TAN PIEN**

Same as Form 5, Figures 12, 13

Hold weight firmly on right leg with its bent knee. Draw left foot with loose ankle close to right without touching floor. Then move left leg backward to southwest diagonal in the Walking Step Space. Straighten left knee and place foot parallel to right foot. Weight is on right bent leg and body is on diagonal slant toward northeast. As left leg moves, move left arm, with palm toward face, in a downward curve in toward body, waist high. Left palm is toward the face; arm is curved. Right arm does not move. (Figure 12)

Continue moving left arm up and outward toward northwest, and then pivoting on left heel, turn toes to point northwest. Place weight on left leg and bend knee to equal bend of right knee. Now your weight is even on both legs. Body is turned northwest. As left foot moves, turn left palm to face northwest. Now both arms are at same level, with wrists slightly higher than shoulder level. Right arm is extended toward northeast, left arm is extended northwest, and left palm faces northwest. (Figure 13)

Movements for Head and Eyes for Form 31

Same as Form 5, Figures 12, 13

Look at left palm. Keep looking at it as hand moves to northwest. Turn head from right to left side, but do *not* bend head downward when eyes look downward. The top of head is kept level as head moves from right to left side. On last movement of left hand to northwest position, look at back of left hand. Left arm, left leg, eyes, and torso move together. (Figures 12, 13)

Form 32. Cloud Arms **YÜN SHOU**

Do not move right arm. Turn left toes inward to north and then move left heel outward to make left foot parallel with right foot. With movements of left foot, shift weight onto right leg and straighten left knee; body slants to northeast. At the same time as you move left foot and shift weight, circle left arm downward and then inward to body waist high, keeping wrist bent. Gradually straightening wrist, move left arm upward toward right wrist. Place left fingers near right pulse, with palm inward facing you. As left arm moves, raise right hand slowly upward, opening hand to face palm northeast. Left foot, left arm, and right hand all move together. (Figure 62)

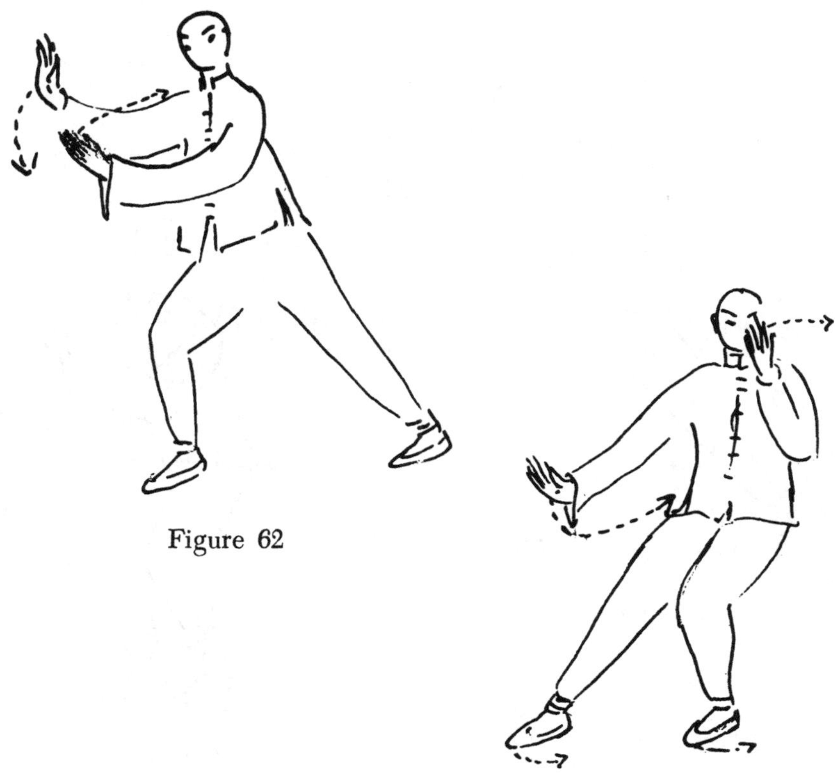

Figure 62

Figure 63

Shift weight back onto left leg, bending left knee and straightening right knee. Feel as if you were sitting on left leg. Torso is erect; back is straight. As weight shifts, move both arms at the same time. Looking at left palm, move left arm to left side, with palm at eye level—twelve inches away from face. Keep eyes fixed on palm. At the same time, circle right arm outward to right side, and then downward, with bent wrist and palm facing down. (Figure 63)

Keeping weight on left leg, turn right toes inward to point northwest. Then turn left toes outward to point northwest. As feet move, torso moves to face northwest. At the same time, both arms move: continue to move left arm, face high, to left side with

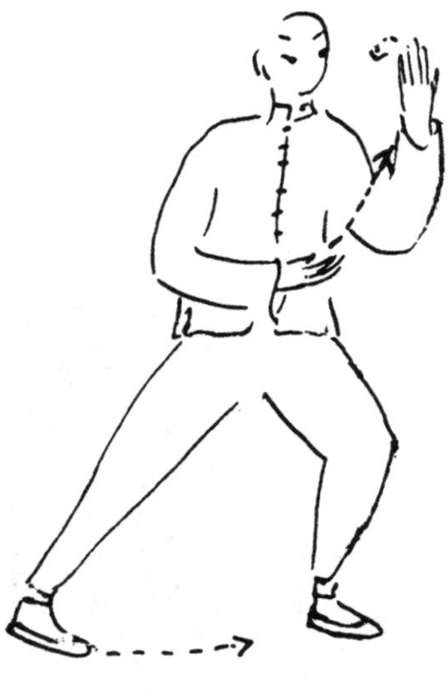

Figure 64

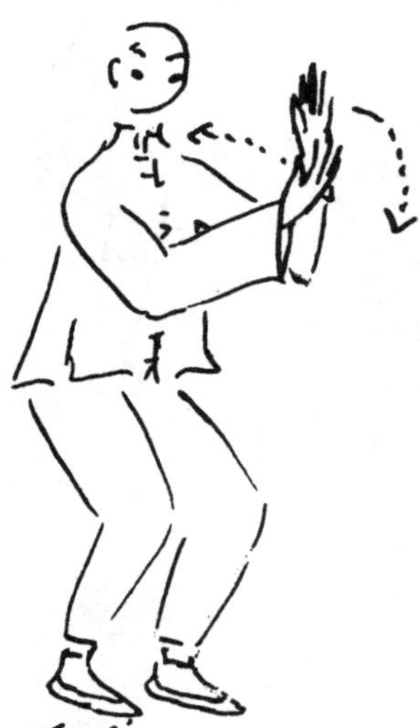

Figure 65

eyes looking at palm. Continue to move right arm in its circle, from downward to inward waist high in front of body, gradually straightening wrist. Then move hand up toward left hand. (Figure 64)

Keeping weight on left leg, place right foot parallel and apart from left in your basic stance: both toes point northwest, both knees are evenly bent, and back is straight. Torso faces northwest. Both arms continue to move: turn left palm to face northwest, at eye level, while you move right fingers up to left pulse, turning right palm toward your face. Look at right palm. Both elbows point downward. (Figure 65)

Turn torso toward right to face northeast, and move right arm to right side, with palm at eye level, twelve inches away from face. Eyes are looking at right palm. Then turn right toes to northeast, placing weight on right leg with its bent knee. Then turn left knee inward, touching left toes to floor, with loose ankle, thus taking weight off left foot. At the same time as right arm and torso turn to northeast, move left arm: circle left arm with palm down and wrist bent outward to left side and then downward. Continue to circle left arm inward waist high in front of body, gradually straightening wrist. Then move it up toward right pulse. (Figure 66)

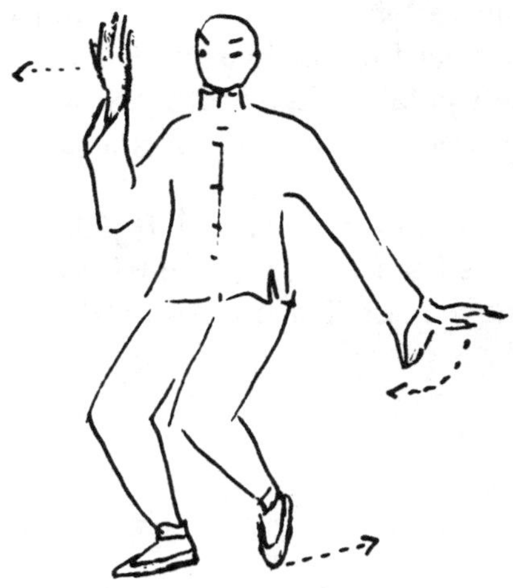

Figure 66

As the left hand goes up toward the right side, place left leg diagonally backward to southwest, in the Walking Step Space. Straighten left knee and bend right knee more deeply with weight on right leg. Body slants to northeast. On this last movement, turn right palm out to face northeast, and place left fingers at right pulse with palm toward face. At this moment eyes look far away toward the northeast. Left hand, right hand, left leg movement, and shifting eye gaze are all made at the same time. (Figure 62)

Repeat Cloud Arms—Figures 63, 64, 65, 66, and 62—again in exactly the same way. *Do not omit this repeat* (see page 13).

Form 33. The Single Whip **TAN PIEN**

Same as Form 5, Figures 12, 13

Continue this from the repeat of Figure 62. Bend right wrist downward and place fingers in Grasping position.

Then move left arm downward and in toward the body waist high; then upward to northwest. (Figure 12)

Turn left palm to face northwest and at the same time turn left toes to point northwest; bend left knee even with right knee. Back is straight.

As left arm moves, look at left palm as it moves downward and upward. Move head from right to left side. Look at back of left hand on its last movement. Torso faces northwest. (Figure 13)

SERIES III

Form 34. On Right—High Pat the Horse KAO T'AN MA

Keeping weight on right leg, move right toes inward to northwest; then move right heel outward to east, and straighten left knee, keeping left foot on floor. This movement on right foot turns torso to west. At the same time as you move right foot, bend right elbow downward and raise right hand upward, opening hand. Then bring hand inward toward right shoulder with palm west. Left palm now faces west. (Figure 67)

Weight remains on right leg with its bent knee. Draw left foot with loose ankle back and place it close to right foot; touch toes to floor. Back is straight. At the same time, both arms move: turning left palm upward, draw left arm inward, while left elbow goes to left side at hip height. Palm is up with straight wrist. Move right arm to west with palm turned to south; keep elbow high so that hand is at face level. Right elbow is bent almost at a right angle. Left palm is level with right elbow. Arms are separated by width of body. (Figure 68)

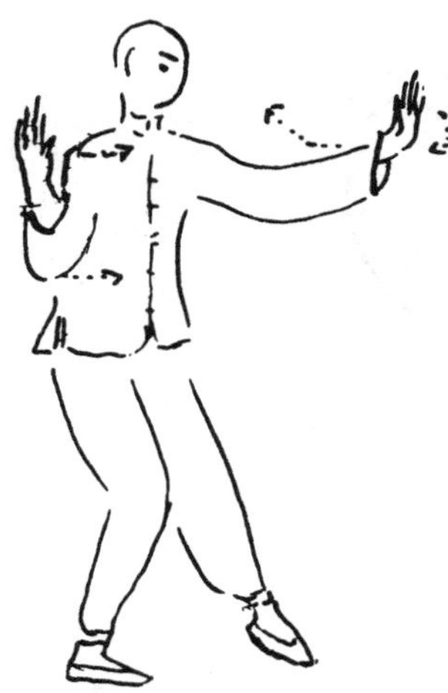

Figure 67

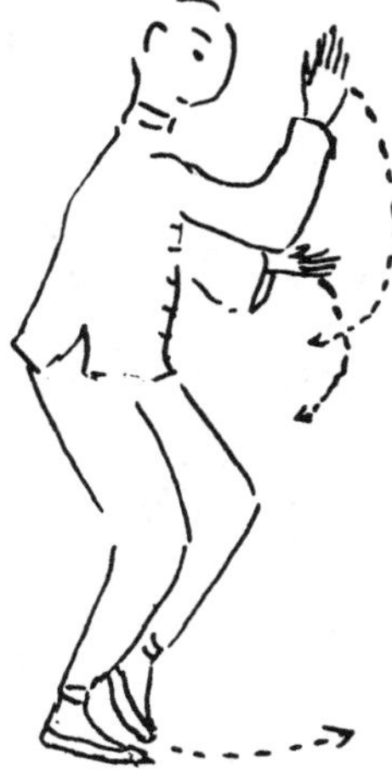

Figure 68

Form 35. On Left—Open Body TSO P'I SHEN

Place left heel forward west in the Walking Step Space; then transfer weight onto left leg, bending left knee and straightening right knee. Body is on a slant toward west. At the same time, both arms move: turn both palms down and move both hands downward toward the center, abdomen high. Right hand goes above the left hand; wrists are crossed; right fingers point southwest; left fingers point northwest. Arms are on a perpendicular. (Figure 69)

Do not move body, legs, or head for next sequence.

Both arms move together making vertical circles: circle left arm downward, then outward to south, then upward to shoulder level, turning palm to face west with fingers pointing south. Then bend left elbow at shoulder level, and bring left hand, making a

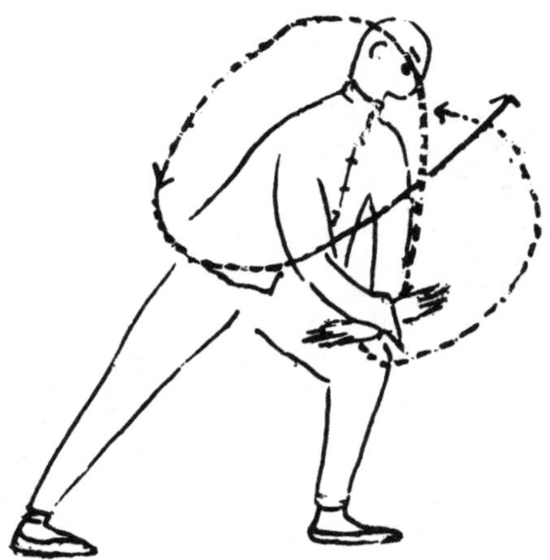

Figure 69

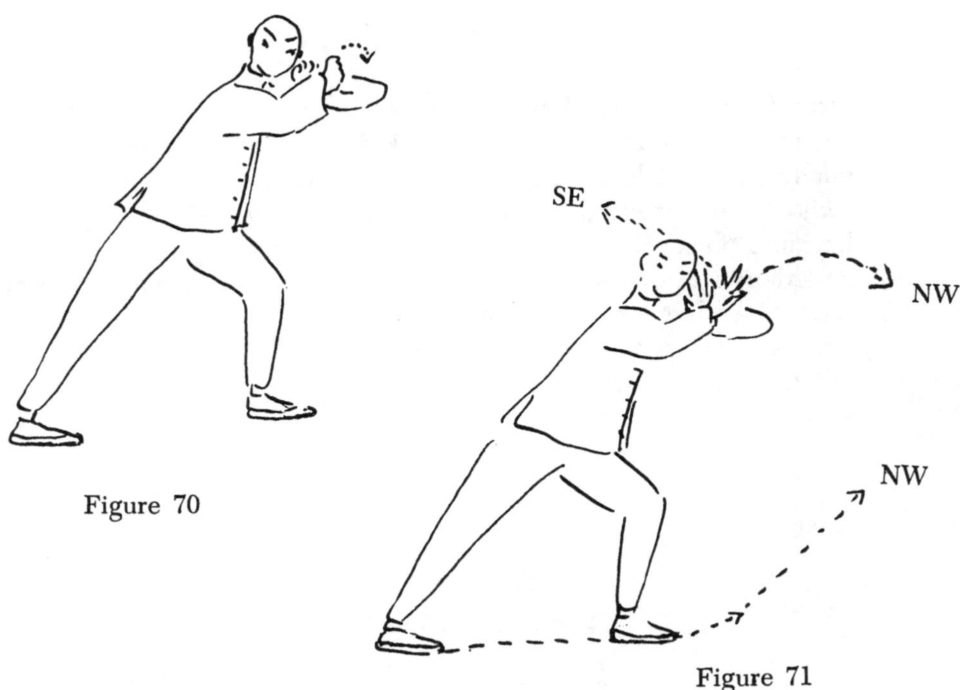

Figure 70

Figure 71

fist of it, to left ear: wrist is straight and fist-palm faces west. At the same time, right arm moves: bring right arm upward as high as forehead with palm up; then move it outward toward north with palm north and fingers up; then downward, turning palm and straightening wrist, in toward body; then up over toward left side, making a fist of right hand, and finally bring it in front of left fist. Wrist-pulses face each other, without touching. Right elbow, in horizontal plane with left elbow, points west. Both wrists side-bend up so that knuckles point upward. (Figure 70)

Then turn head to look north. Do not tilt head. (Figure 70)

Now turn right fist-palm to face west. Then open both hands spreading fingers very wide apart from each other. Direct fingers to point to ceiling; do not move elbows. Legs and torso and head have remained still. (Figure 71)

Form 36. Raise Right Leg T'I YU CHIAO

Draw right foot with loose ankle close to left foot, without touching floor. Then raise leg up toward northwest angle. Leg is straight; foot is turned inward, with toes leading (see page 30). At the same time, move both arms: move right arm to shoulder level, toward northwest, with palm facing southwest and with straight wrist. Move left arm curved outward toward southeast: palm faces southeast and is above shoulder level, wrist is bent and fingers point toward ceiling. (Figure 72)

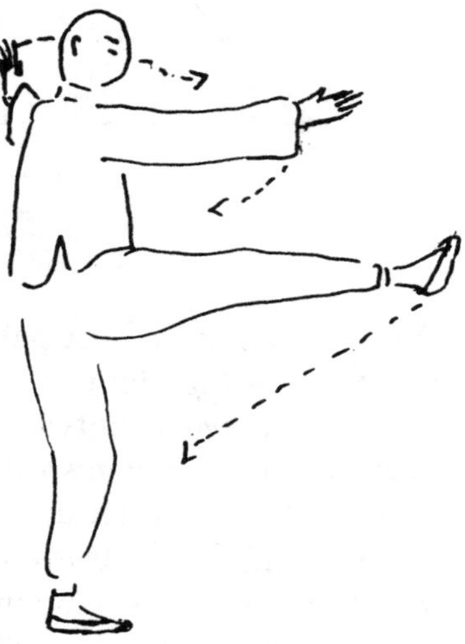

Figure 72

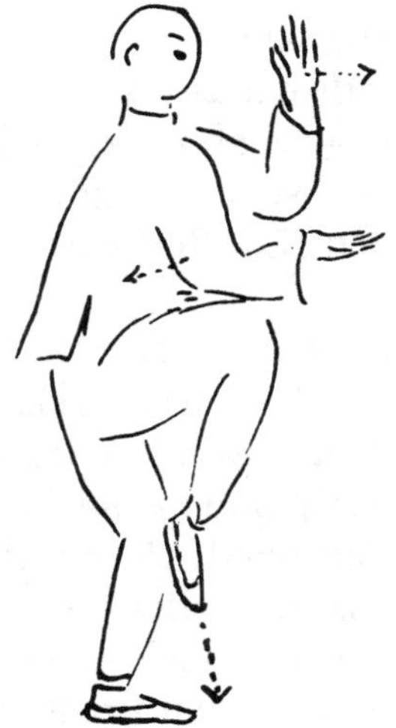

Figure 73

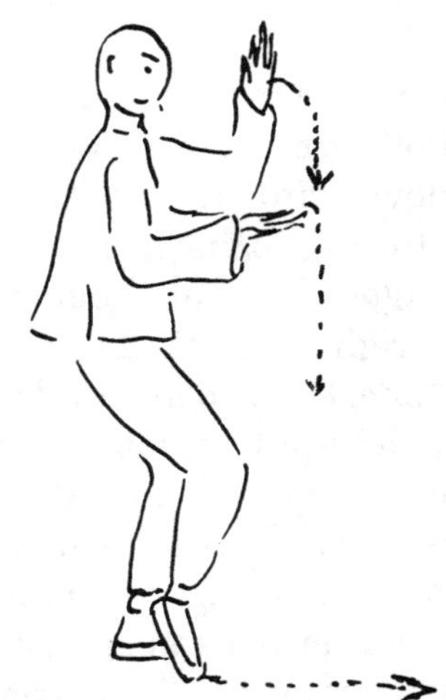

Figure 74

Form 37. On Left—High Pat the Horse KAO T'AN MA

Bend right leg keeping knee high. Then bring foot with loose ankle close to left knee. At the same time, draw both arms inward, each toward its shoulder, by bending both elbows. Right elbow is lower than left. (Figure 73)

Bending left knee, place right toes on floor lightly. At the same time, both arms move into position: turn right palm upward and left palm north; then move left arm toward west with palm north, keeping left elbow high so that hand is at face level. Left elbow is bent almost at a right angle. Right elbow goes near right hip; right palm is level with left elbow, and arms are separated by width of body. (Figure 74)

Form 38. On Right—Open Body YU P'I SHEN

Reverse of Figures 69, 70, 71

Place right heel forward west in the Walking Step space; then transfer weight onto right leg, bending knee and straightening left knee. Body is on a slant forward west. At the same time, both arms move: turn both palms down and move both hands downward toward the center, abdomen high. Left hand goes above right hand, wrists are crossed, left fingers point northwest, and right fingers point southwest. Arms are on a perpendicular. (Reverse of Figure 69)

Do not move body, legs, or head for next sequence.

Both arms move together making vertical circles: circle right arm downward, then outward to north, then upward to shoulder level, turning palm to face west with fingers pointing north. Then bend right elbow at shoulder level and bring hand, closing it to a fist, to right ear. Wrist is straight and fist-palm faces west. At the same time, left arm moves: bring left arm upward as high as forehead with palm up; then move it outward toward south with palm south and fingers upward; then downward, turning palm and straightening wrist in toward body; then up over toward right side making a fist of left hand and bringing it in front of right fist. Wrist-pulses face each other and do not touch. Left elbow in horizontal plane with right elbow points west. Both wrists side-bend up so that knuckles point upward. (Reverse of Figure 70)

Then turn head to look south. Do not tilt head. (Reverse of Figure 70)

Now turn left fist-palm to face west. Open both hands, spreading fingers very wide apart from each other. Direct fingers to point to ceiling; do not move elbows. Legs and torso and head have remained still. (Figure 71)

Form 39. Raise Left Leg T'I TSO CHIAO

Draw left foot, with loose ankle, close to right foot, not touching floor. Then raise leg up toward southwest angle. Leg is straight; foot is turned inward, with toes leading (see page 30). At the same time, both arms move: move left arm at shoulder level toward the southwest, palm facing northwest, with wrist straight. Move right arm curved outward toward northeast: palm faces northeast and is above shoulder level; wrist is bent, and fingers point toward ceiling. (Figure 75)

Form 40. Pivot Body on Heel—Raise Leg

CHUAN SHEN TENG CHIAO

Bend left knee, keeping it high. Move leg so that knee points west, and place left foot with loose ankle close to right knee: left foot is turned inward (see page 30). At the same time, both arms move: make a fist of right hand and bring it near right ear with elbow at shoulder level, pointing north. Make fist of left hand and bring it in front of right wrist, with pulses facing each other. Elbow is same height as right elbow. Head does not move: it faces south; weight is on right leg. (Figure 76)

Keep arms and head in position. Pivot on right heel, turning body to face south by placing right toes to point directly south. Head

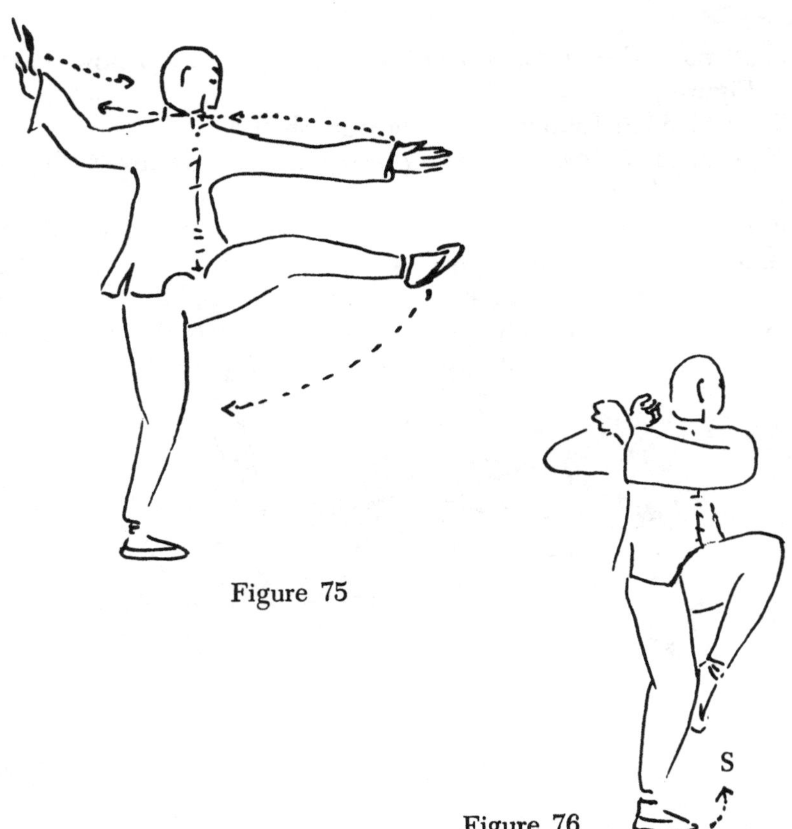

Figure 75

Figure 76

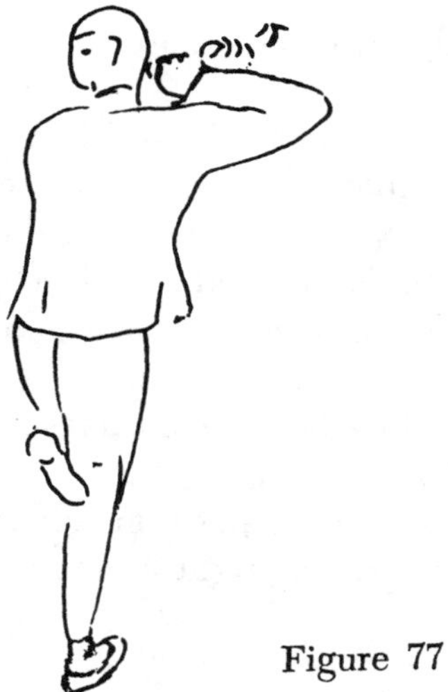

Figure 77

looks east now. Fists remain near right ear; right elbow now points west. (Figure 77)

Then turn left fist outward to face south.

Now open both hands and spread fingers wide apart, fingers pointing to ceiling.

Raise left leg directly to east and flex foot (see page 30). At the same time, both arms move: move right arm to west, so that hand with wrist bent is above shoulder level: palm is west and fingers point up. Move left arm to east shoulder high: palm faces south with fingers east, and wrist is straight. (Figure 78)

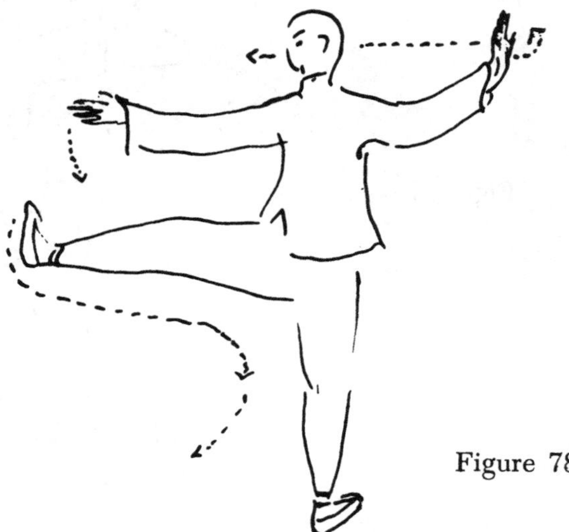

Figure 78

Form 41. Brush Knee and Twist Step LOU HSI NIU PU

Draw left leg inward to body, keeping knee high, and place foot with loose ankle near right knee. Bend more deeply on right knee and turn torso to face east. Straightening left knee, place left heel on floor to east in direct line with right heel: weight is on right leg with its bent knee. At the same time, both arms move: bending right elbow downward, draw right hand inward toward right shoulder. As torso shifts to face east, palm faces to east. Bring left arm, with palm south, halfway downward toward left side. (Figure 79)

Shift weight onto left leg, bending its knee and straightening right knee. Body is on a slant toward east. At the same time, both arms continue their movements: bring right arm forward east in line with right shoulder: palm faces east and wrist is bent. Move left arm downward to left side of left thigh, with wrist straight and palm facing thigh. Turn the heel of right foot to west as you move both arms. Now feet are parallel and are in the Walking Step position. (Figure 80)

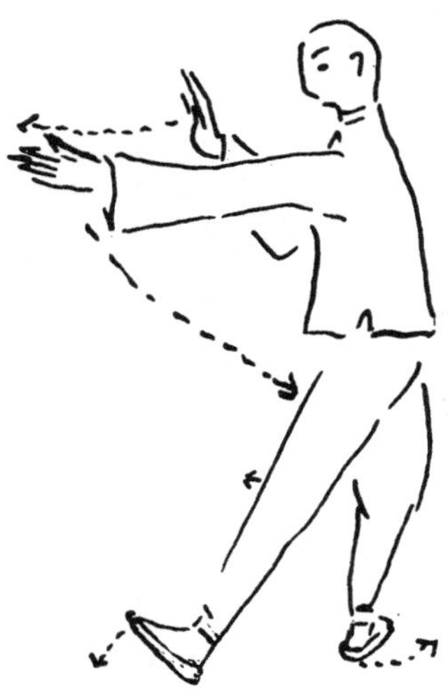

Figure 79

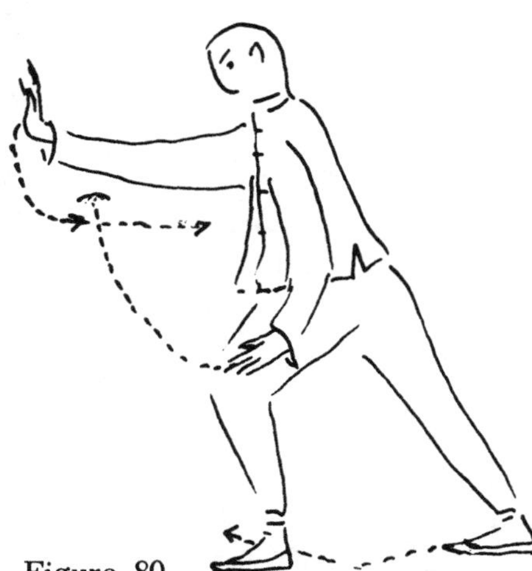

Figure 80

Form 42. Plant Leg and Punch Step CHIN PU TSAI CH'UI

Draw right leg with loose ankle close to left foot, not touching floor. Left knee is bent; weight is on left leg. Both arms move at the same time as right leg moves; circle right arm inward toward center: fingers point north and palm faces east. Move left hand up over right wrist, with fingers pointing to east.

Continue moving arms: circle right hand under left; make a fist of it, turning fist-palm upward. Draw fist toward right hip, with elbow pointing to west, and begin to move left hand, with palm south, to east, in line with left shoulder. (Figure 81)

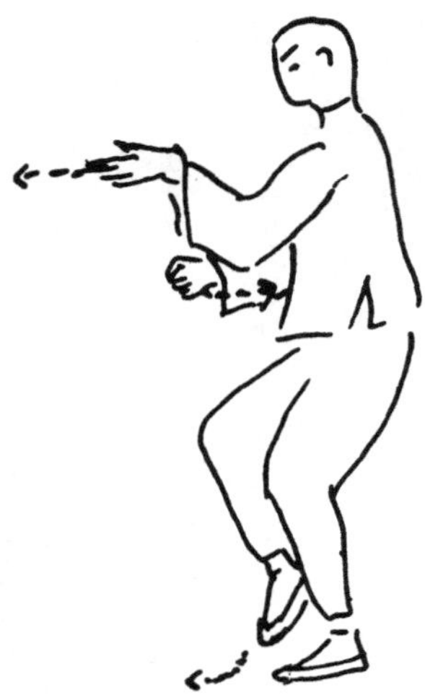

Figure 81

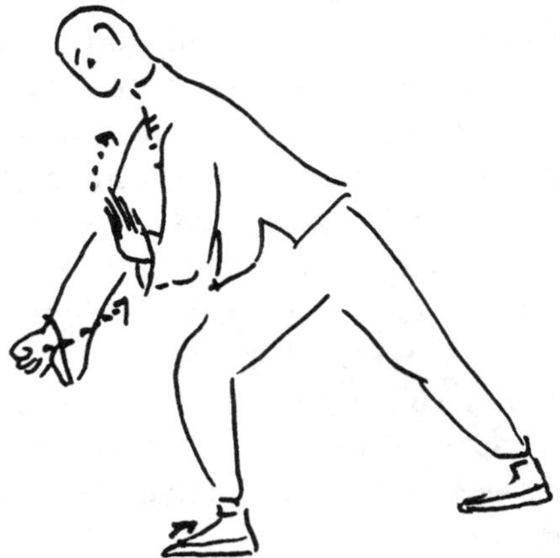

Figure 82

Step forward east quickly on right foot; then *quickly* step forward east on left foot, bending its knee and straightening right knee. Weight is forward on left: body slants on a diagonal and bends downward. This rhythm is extremely quick—like a flash, moving with a quick step from right to left foot. (Figure 82)

As you step quickly forward on right leg, both arms also move quickly: pull right fist to right hip and push left arm outward toward east (similar to the gesture of stretching a bow open to shoot an arrow).

Then as you step quickly onto left foot, punch right fist toward east, diagonally downward. At the same time, move left palm to inner right elbow, bending wrist with fingers upward; elbow is bent. This punch is done with hard force. Keep heel of right foot on floor. (Figure 82)

Form 43. Turn Body—Throw Fist TAN SHEN P'IEH SHEN CH'UI

Keeping weight on left leg, raise torso to an upright position. At the same time, both arms move: bring left palm up to face right shoulder; bend right elbow, and bring forearm up to cross left forearm, so that right fist-palm faces left shoulder. Both elbows point downward; right arm is on the outer side of this cross. (Figure 83)

While you are moving torso and both arms into position, start the Toe-Heel-Heel Step (page 31). Turn toes of left foot inward to point south. Then turn right heel inward making feet parallel, with weight remaining on left leg: now body faces south. Then turn left heel outward to east; weight is still on left. Now torso faces southwest. Then raise right toes off floor, with right heel touching floor lightly. Now body faces west. (Figure 84)

While you are raising right toes off floor and turning to face west, both hands move: turn hands to face west; moving them to center of chest, place left palm behind right fist, spreading left fingers wide apart. (Figure 84)

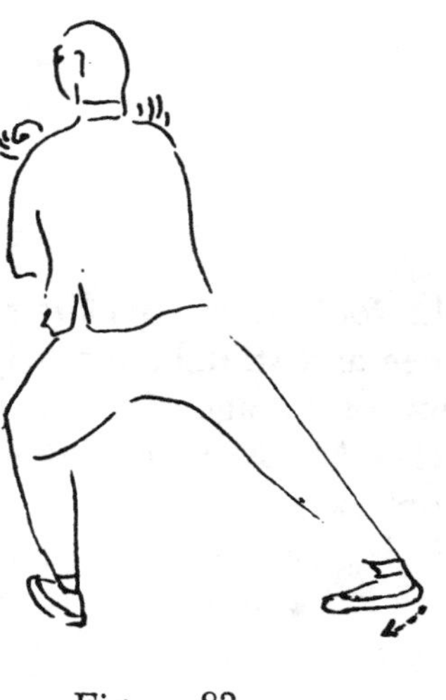

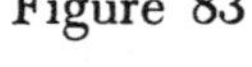

Figure 83

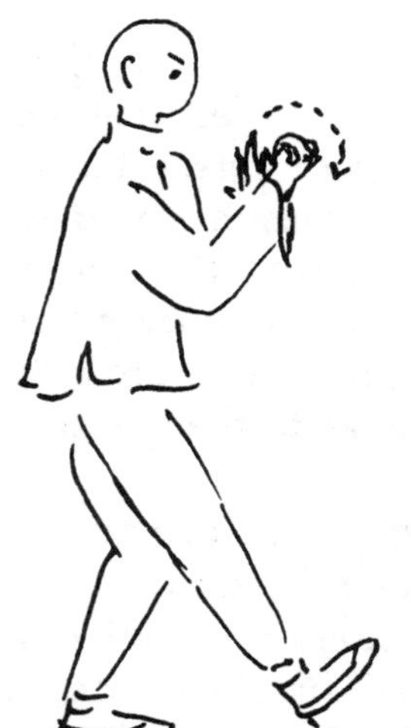

Figure 84

Form 44. On Right—High Pat the Horse KAO T'AN MA

Same as Form 34, Figure 68

Place right heel forward in the Walking Step Space; transfer weight onto right leg, bending its knee and straightening left knee. At the same time, move left hand over right fist in a small circle. Place weight on right leg with its bent knee, and draw left toes with loose ankle close to right foot, touching floor. At the same time, turning left palm up, move left arm downward and place elbow near left hip. Move right arm outward west with palm to south: right elbow and left palm are at same level. Arms are separated by the width of body. (Figure 68)

Form 45. On Left—Open Body TSO P'I SHEN

Same as Form 35, Figures 69, 70, 71

Place left heel forward west in the Walking Step Space; then transfer weight onto left leg, bending knee and straightening right knee. Body is on a slant toward west. At the same time, both arms move: turn both palms down and move both hands downward toward the center, abdomen high. Right hand goes above left hand; wrists are crossed; right fingers point southwest; left fingers point northwest. Both arms are on a perpendicular. (Figure 69)

Do not move body, legs, or head for the next sequence.

Both arms move together making vertical circles: circle left arm downward, then outward toward south, then up to shoulder level, turning palm to face west, with fingers pointing south. Then bend left elbow at shoulder level and bring left hand, closing to a fist, to left ear; wrist is straight and fist-palm faces west. At the same time, right arm moves: bring right arm upward with palm facing up, as high as forehead; then move it outward toward north with palm north and fingers up, then downward, turning palm and straightening wrist,toward body; then up over toward left side, making a fist of right hand and bringing it in front of left fist. Wrist-pulses face each other without touching. Right elbow is in horizontal plane with left elbow and points west. Both wrists side-bend up so that knuckles point upward. (Figure 70)

Turn head to look north. Do not tilt head. (Figure 70) Turn right fist-palm to face west. Then open both hands, spreading fingers very wide apart from each other. Direct fingers to point to ceiling. Do not move elbows. Legs and torso and head have remained still. (Figure 71)

Form 46. Raise Right Leg T'I YU CHIAO

Same as Form 38, Figure 72

Draw right foot with loose ankle close to left foot, not touching floor. Then raise right leg toward northwest angle. Leg is straight; foot is turned inward with toes leading. At the same time, both arms move: move right arm, at shoulder level, toward northwest so that palm faces southwest with straight wrist. Move left arm curved outward toward southeast: palm faces southeast and is above shoulder level; wrist is bent and fingers point toward ceiling. (Figure 72)

Form 47. Retreat Step—Beat the Tiger T'UI PU TA HU

Weight is on left leg. Bend right knee and bring right foot with loose ankle inward toward left knee. At the same time, torso and left arm move: bend left elbow downward and turn palm to face northwest, moving hand to left shoulder. As arm moves, turn torso to face northwest. (Figure 85)

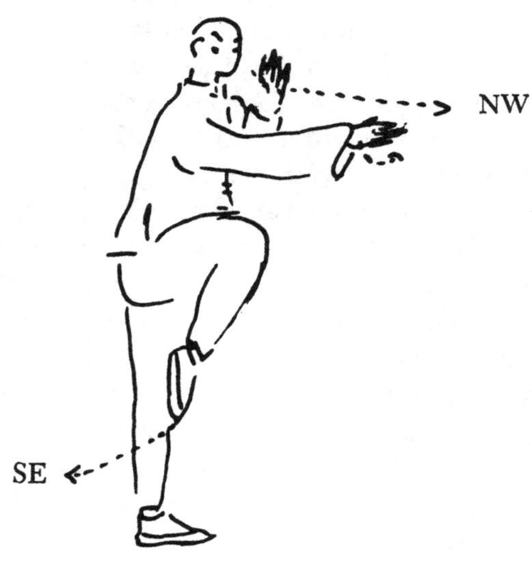

Figure 85

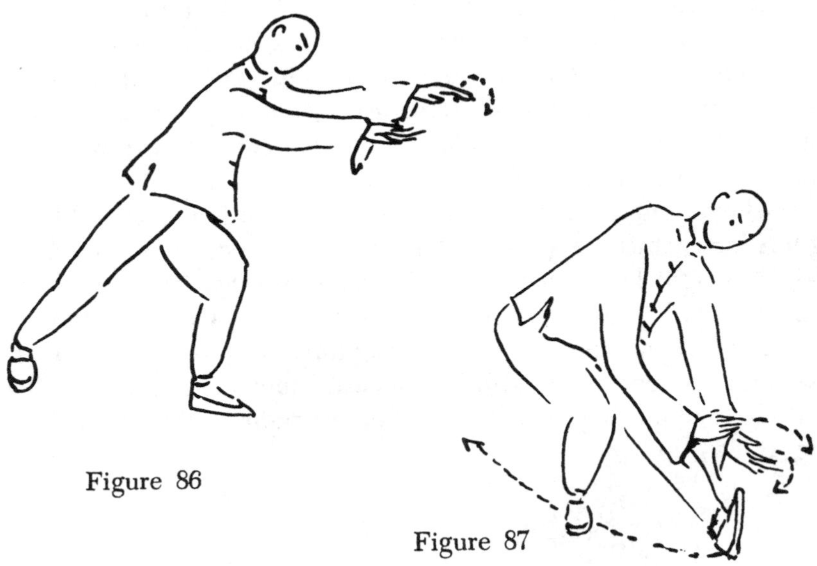

Figure 86

Figure 87

Bend left knee, lowering body, and place right foot diagonally backward toward southeast, straightening right knee: place right foot so that toes point north. Weight remains on left leg with its bent knee. Body is on a slant diagonally toward the northwest; left toes are pointing west. At the same time as right leg moves, move both arms: move left arm facing palm down toward northwest, in line with left shoulder. Pulling right shoulder back a bit, turn right palm to face up; elbows and wrists are straight. Fingers of both hands point northwest. (Figure 86)

Shift weight back onto right bending right knee and straighten left knee, and flexing left foot which is therefore angled upward toward west. As you sit back and shift weight onto right leg, bend torso forward and downward over left leg. Move both arms at the same time as legs and torso move: turn left palm up and turn right palm down; place right fingers at left pulse, angling right hand so that it is at right angles to left arm. Right elbow is up, and left elbow is down. Left arm is straight and parallel to left leg. Legs, torso, and arms move together. (Figure 87)

Keeping body low, move right hand in a small horizontal circle over left hand, while turning left palm to face floor and gradually making hands into fists. Finish circle movement so that fists are about ten inches apart, just above right foot. In the meantime, left leg moves: keeping weight on right leg with its bent knee, move left leg diagonally toward southeast, straightening knee, and place left foot with toes pointing west. Both fists get into place above right foot as left foot arrives in its place. Body is bent forward over right bent leg. Do not drop head. (Figure 88)

Swing both arms and torso from right side to left side, and bending left knee, shift weight onto left leg. Turn right toes inward and straighten right knee, then turn left toes to southwest. Now weight is on left leg. Fists and torso now are near left leg. Continue to move torso: twist at left side of waist, moving torso back to east; gradually raise torso and both arms, still facing east. Move curved left arm upward to shoulder height and bring curved right arm to waist level. (Figure 89)

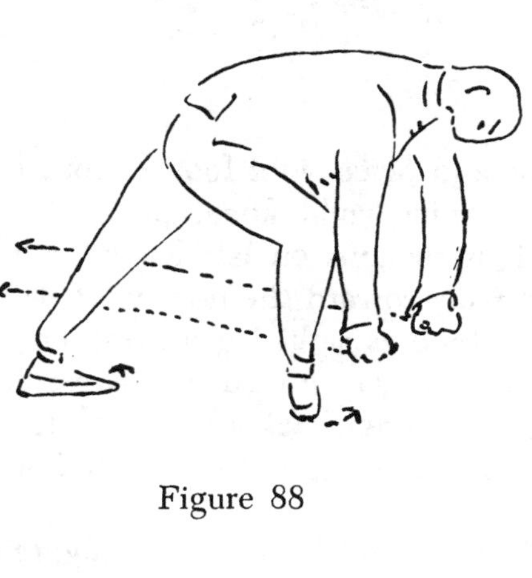

Figure 88

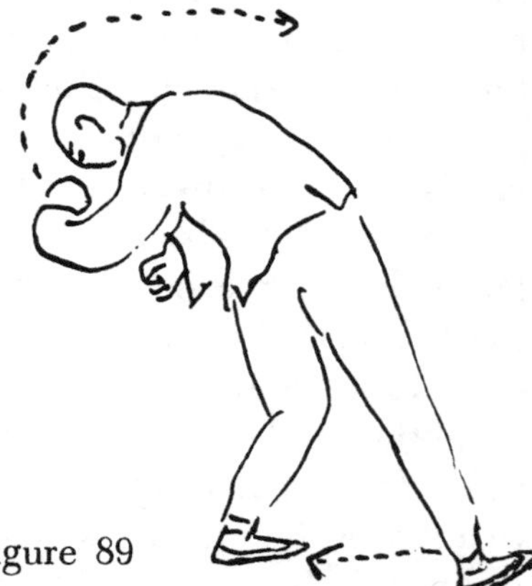

Figure 89

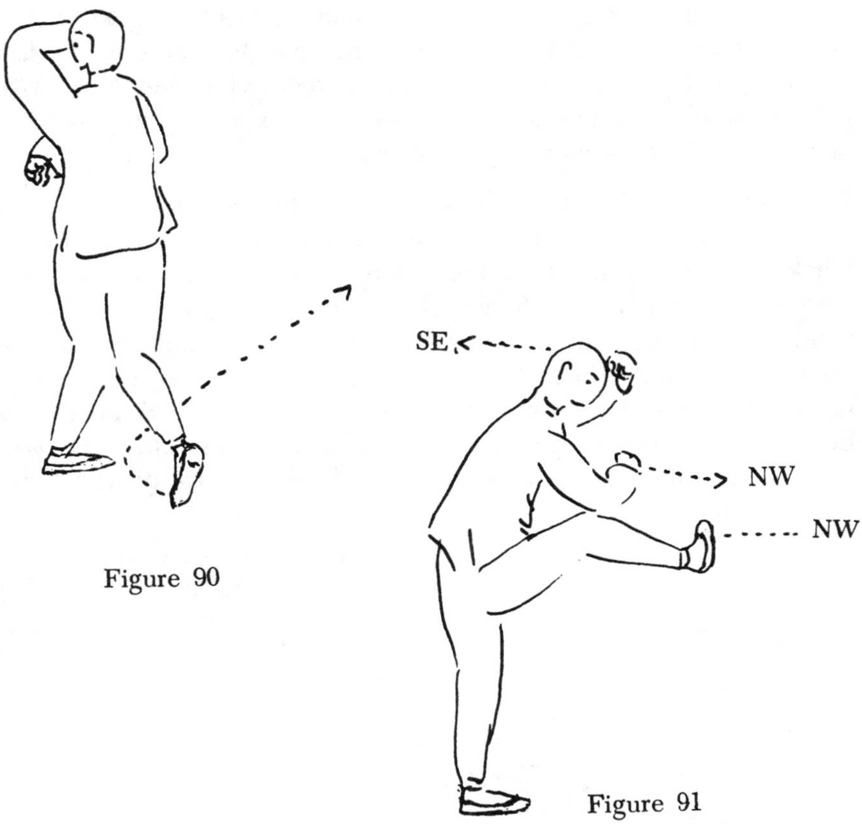

Figure 90

Figure 91

Next lift torso up, erect, and face southeast, bringing left arm in a curve around forehead; keep right arm curved at waist height. As you do this, keeping all weight on left leg with its bent knee, draw right foot with loose ankle to left foot. (Figure 90)

Continue to turn torso: move torso to face south and then to face west. At the same time, raise right leg so that it is directed to west; flex foot. Knee is high and bent, with lower leg held high. As right leg lifts, bend body slightly forward over right leg. Touch right elbow to right knee: right arm is curved waist high with fist-palm facing inward to body. Left arm is curved around forehead with fist-palm facing outward. The whole body is directed to west. (Figure 91)

Form 48. Open—Extend Right Leg YU FEN CHIAO

Extend right leg to northwest angle, straightening knee and keeping foot flexed. At the same time, move right arm, opening fist, above right leg and touch toes with fingers, while left arm, with palm to southeast, moves to southeast: fingers are up and wrist is bent. Torso does not move. (Figure 92)

Form 49. Strike Ears with Fists SHUANG FENG KUAN ERH

Bend right knee and bring right foot with loose ankle close to left knee. Bending left knee more deeply, place right heel forward west in the Walking Step Space; then transfer weight onto right leg, bending its knee, and straighten left knee: body slants forward to west. At the same time, move both arms inward toward the forehead with palms facing west. Place hands near forehead, finger tips pointing to each other; palms face west. Elbows point outward, right to north and left to south. Hands are a fist-length away from forehead. (Figure 93)

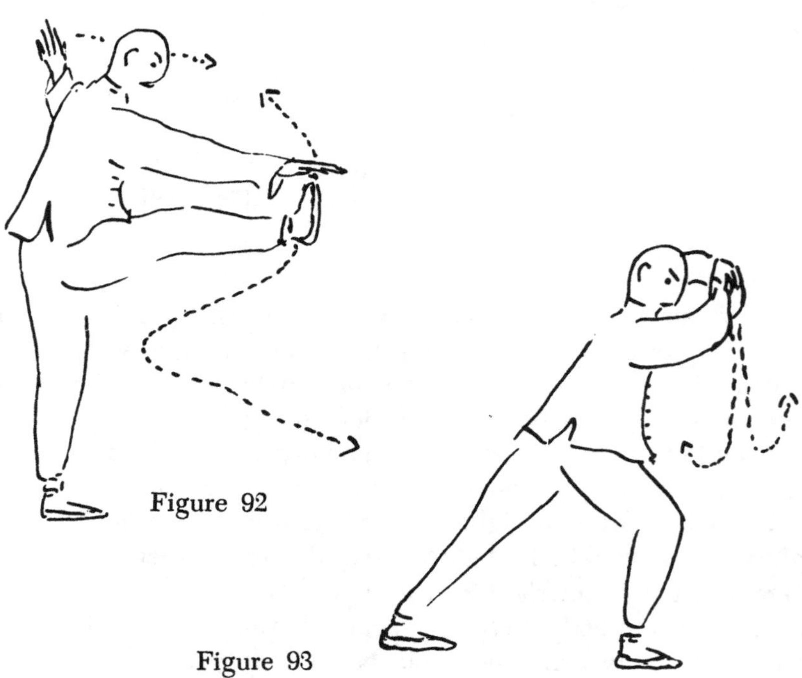

Figure 92

Figure 93

Do not move legs, torso, or head. Move both arms downward vertically, in front of body: palms face floor, wrists are bent, and arms are curved. Move arms in opposite directions, keeping fingers pointing inward and wrists bent: move right arm outward to north, and move left outward to south, then up to shoulder level. Bend elbows, keeping palms west, and bring hands to center of forehead, making fists of them. Arms have described a vertical circle. Fists are a fist-length away from forehead. (Figure 93, except that hands are now fisted.)

Form 50. Turn Body—Open Body FAN SHEN YU P'I SHEN

Weight is on right leg with bent knee. Turn toes of right foot to point north, and twist torso to face north. Pull right elbow to right side, east, in line with right shoulder; place right fist near right ear. With movement of right arm, move left arm over to right side and place left wrist in front of right wrist. Fist-palms face each other. Head remains looking west. Right toes, torso, and arms move and finish at the same time. (Figure 94)

Turn left fist-palm to face north. Then open hands, spreading fingers very wide apart, and direct fingers to point to ceiling.

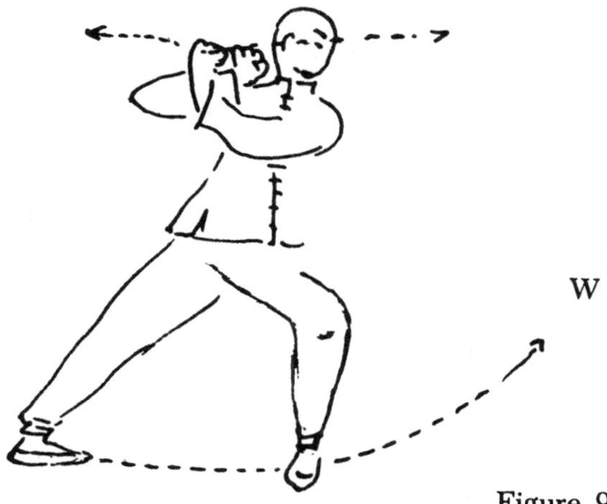

Figure 94

Form 51. Raise the Left Leg T'I TSO CHIAO

Draw left foot with loose ankle to right foot; then raise left leg directly to west with straightened knee and flexed foot. On leg movement, separate arms: move left arm to west shoulder high, with wrist straight and palm north. Move right arm to east, bending wrist and turning palm to face east with fingers pointing toward ceiling. (Figure 95)

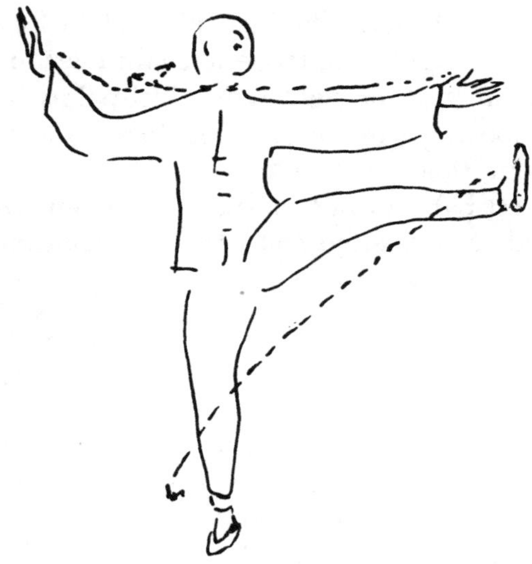

Figure 95

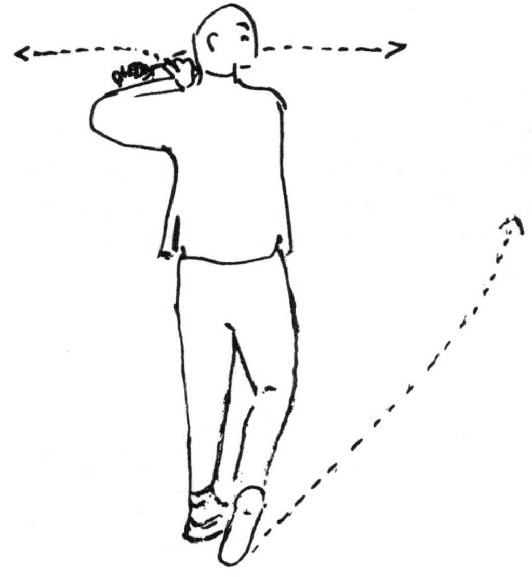

Figure 96

Form 52. Turn the Body—Open Body FAN SHEN TSO Pʻ I SHEN

Swing left leg around right leg *quickly* pivoting on right foot, and turning to face south. Place left foot in front of—therefore to the south ~~of~~—right foot. All this is done quickly. Adjust weight firmly on left foot: left toes to point south, left knee is straight, and right knee is bent, with right heel *off* ground, and toes touching floor. As you make this quick turn, bend left elbow shoulder high, make a fist of left hand, and bring it to left ear; at the same time, bend right elbow, make a right fist, and place right wrist in front of left wrist. As you make the quick turn and as you cross your wrists, head turns to look to west. All movements with legs, head, and arms are done as quickly as possible.

Turn right fist-palm to face south. Open hands, spreading fingers very wide and apart; direct fingers to point to ceiling. While you are moving hands, fix weight firmly on left leg so that right leg is free to move. (Figure 96)

Form 53. Raise the Right Leg T'I YU CHIAO

Raise right leg directly to west with straightened knee and flexed foot. With this leg movement, separate arms: move right arm to west shoulder high, with wrist straight and palm south; move left arm to east, bending wrist and turning palm to east with fingers pointing toward ceiling. (Figure 97)

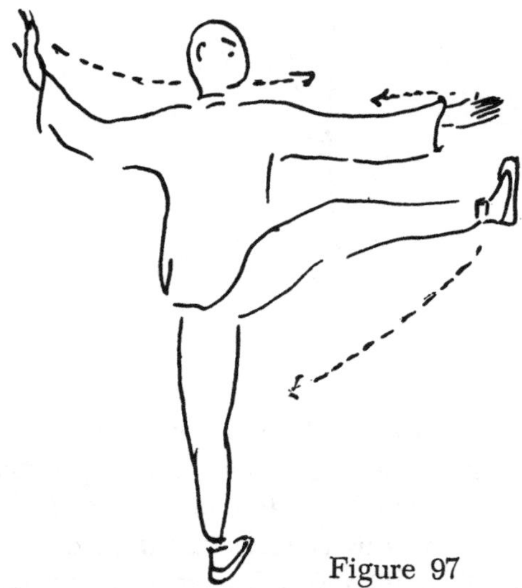

Figure 97

Form 54. Step Up, Parry, and Punch CHIN PU PAN LAN CH'UI

Same as Form 12, Figures 28, 29, 30

Bend right knee and bring right foot with loose ankle near left knee. Bend on left knee more deeply. At the same time move both arms inward toward body; bend left elbow downward and bring hand near shoulder with palm to west; bend right elbow down and face palm south. Keep right hand in line with right shoulder. (Figure 98)

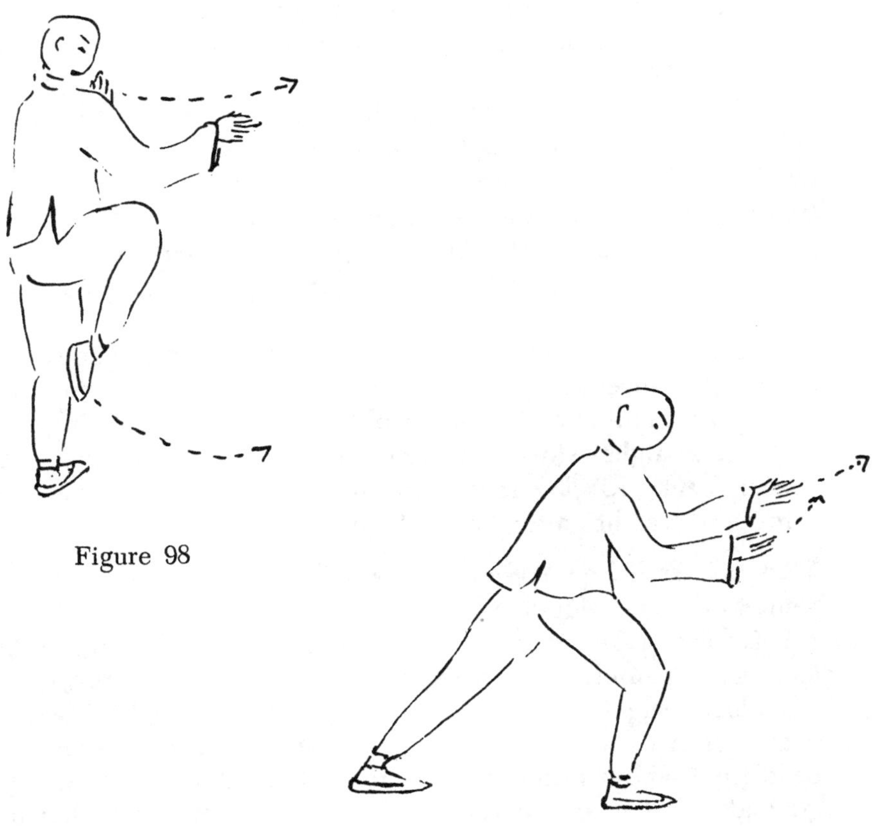

Figure 98

Figure 99

With weight on left leg with its bent knee, place right heel forward west in the Walking Step Space; then transfer weight onto right leg, bending its knee, and straightening left knee. At the same time, move left heel outward to make foot parallel to right foot. Move both arms at the same time as leg moves: move left arm forward west in line with left shoulder, with palm to north; and begin to move right arm forward west, with palm south. (Figure 99)

Move left foot with loose ankle close to right foot. Then place heel forward west in the Walking Step Space, and transfer weight onto left leg bending its knee and straightening right knee. Body is on a slant forward west. At the same time, continue to move arms: bring right arm forward and place fingertips near left pulse; bend left hand so that fingers point west-downward, with palm north. (Figure 28)

Shift weight back onto right leg, bending right knee, straightening left knee, and flexing foot. At the same time, both arms move: draw right hand close along left forearm toward its elbow and then bring right hand down toward right hip, gradually making a fist of it. Right elbow points to north; fist-palm is turned upward. While right arm moves, angle left hand so that fingers point upward-west. (Figure 29)

Shift weight forward onto left leg, bending its knee and straightening right knee. At the same time, both arms move: move right arm up west in line with right shoulder, with fist-palm facing south: elbow is straight. Move left palm near inner side of right elbow: wrist is bent with fingers pointing to ceiling. Arm movements and shifting of weight go together. (Figure 30)

Form 55. As If You Were Shutting a Door JU FENG SZU PI

Same as Form 13, Figures 31, 32

Do not move legs or torso. Move left hand under right arm to its outer side, and turn palm to face right elbow. (Figure 31)

Shift weight back onto right leg, bending right knee, and straighten left knee, flexing foot. At the same time, both arms move: bend right elbow, bringing fist in toward left shoulder, opening fist gradually so that right palm faces left shoulder, and move left palm facing inward, in to face right shoulder. Left arm is on the outside of right arm. Both elbows are bent downward and forearms are crossed on a diagonal.

At the same time both arms move: move right hand in front of right shoulder with palm facing it and move left hand in front of left shoulder with palm facing it. Elbows are bent downward, wrists are straight, and fingers point to ceiling.

Next, turn both palms to face west, keeping wrists straight and elbows down. All these arm movements are made as weight is shifted from left back onto right leg with bent knee. (Figure 32)

Form 56. Carry Tiger, Push Mountain PAO HU T'UI SHAN

Same as Form 14, Figures 33, 34

Shift weight forward onto left leg, bending knee and straightening right knee. At the same time, push both hands, which are facing west, forward shoulder high to west, each arm in line with its shoulder: wrists are shoulder high; body slants forward on a diagonal west. (Figure 33)

Keep weight on left leg. Bend torso forward and down, moving arms at same time; lower arms so that palms face floor at knee level. Arms are perpendicular to floor. (Figure 34)

Form 57. Cross Hands SHIH TSU SHOU

Same as Form 15, Figures 35, 36, 37

Turn right toes to north and at the same time, shift weight onto right leg, bending its knee and straightening left knee. With these movements, torso moves to north, still remaining bent over. At the same time as torso and right toes move, move right hand to right side of right leg, keeping palm facing down: right fingers now point east. Left hand remains at left side; palm is down with fingers pointing west. (Figure 35)

Turn left toes to north, and at the same time gradually raise torso to an upright position, bringing arms up sideways shoulder high. Then move them forward north, shoulder high. Straighten wrists as you raise torso and arms. (Figure 36)

Keeping right knee bent, place left foot parallel to right and apart from it, in your basic stance. Both knees are bent. At the same time, bring both arms inward, crossing forearms diagonally: right forearm is on the outside of left; left palm faces east on a slant, right palm faces west on a slant. The cross of the arms is a little below chin level about twelve inches away from the face. Elbows are high; back is straight. (Figure 37)

Form 58. Oblique Brush Knee Twist Step HSIEH LOU HSI NIU PU

Same as Form 16, to northwest on right side

Move heel of right foot outward to southeast, keeping weight on right leg with its bent knee. This movement releases weight from left leg, and turns torso to face northwest.

Move left leg to northwest, straightening knee and flexing foot. Place left heel in the Walking Step Space. Then transfer weight onto left leg, bending knee and straightening right knee. Body slants forward northwest. At the same time both arms move: move right arm forward northwest in line with right shoulder, turning palm to face northwest, and move left arm with bent wrist downward in front of left thigh; fingers point northwest and palm is down. (Figure 38)

Toe-Heel-Heel-Step
Same as Figures 39–1, 2, 3, 4

Keeping weight on left leg with its bent knee, move left toes inward to point northeast. Straighten torso. At the same time both arms move: move left hand upward with fingers leading, and move right hand inward toward body. (Figure 39–1)

Keeping weight on left leg with its bent knee, move right heel inward, making right foot parallel to left, and bend right knee, so that toes of both feet point northeast. Weight is still on left leg, and torso is straight. At the same time, continue to move both hands toward center of body, with left hand approaching right wrist. (Figure 39–2)

Keeping weight on left leg with its bent knee, move left heel outward to northwest. With this movement torso faces east and right knee straightens. Feet are now in T position. At the same time, arms move: continue to move left hand over right wrist, with left fingers pointing southeast; right wrist is bent. (Figure 39–3)

Weight is still on left leg with its bent knee. Turning torso to face southeast, raise right toes off floor. At the same time, both arms move: move right arm with bent wrist down toward front of right thigh, and move left arm up toward southeast. (Figure 39–4)

Oblique Brush Knee Twist Step
To southeast on left side

Place right heel to southeast in the Walking Step Space. Transfer weight onto right leg, bending knee and straightening left knee. Body slants southeast on a diagonal. At the same time, both arms move: move left arm to southeast in line with left shoulder, turning palm to face southeast, and move right hand down to front of right thigh, with palm facing floor and fingers pointing southeast. (Opposite of Figure 38)

Form 59. Grasping the Bird's Tail LAN CH'ÜEH WEI
Same as Form 17, Figures 7, 8, 9, 10, 11; (first)

Shift weight back onto left leg, bending knee, straightening right knee, and flexing foot. At the same time both arms move: bring right arm up to southeast, chin high, with palm facing northeast, and place left fingers at right pulse. (Figure 7, except that here you face southeast instead of east)

Keep the relationship of hands the same. Bending both elbows downward and slightly out, draw both arms inward toward body at chin level. Do not come too close to your face.

Turn right palm up and left palm down. As hands move, angle left hand so that it is at right angles to right wrist; therefore left elbow points to northeast. (Figure 8, except that here you face southeast)

Grasping the Bird's Tail (second)

Transfer weight onto right leg, bending knee and straightening left knee, with body on a slant to southeast. At the same time as you transfer weight, stretch right arm to east, chin high, straightening elbow. Keep left fingers above right pulse. (Figure 9, except that here you face east.)

Move both arms in a horizontal circle, chin high, from east, to southeast, to south, and to west. When arms reach south, bend right elbow downward and bend wrist so that palm faces upward. Both right and left fingers point west. Left arm is adjusted to movements of right arm, because left fingers remain near right pulse.

As you make circling movement from south to west, shift weight onto left leg, bending its knee, and straighten right, flexing foot. (Figure 10, except here you face southeast)

Grasping the Bird's Tail (third)

Pivot on right heel turning toes to northeast, and place foot on floor. At the same time, raise right arm with palm leading up toward ceiling; circle it over and down to northeast, straightening arm as you do so, and stop at place where right wrist is slightly above shoulder height. (Figure 11)

As you are approaching this last position, bend right knee, placing weight on right leg. At the same time bend right wrist, and lower right hand downward so that fingers point downward. As hand bends down place all fingers close together over the thumb as if grasping it. Right arm remains in its position when wrist bends and fingers move. Left fingers are still at right pulse, with palm toward the face. Left wrist is straight and arm is curved. (Figure 11)

Form 60. The Single Whip TAN PIEN

Same as Form 5, except that here you finish facing *north*, Figures 12, 13

Holding weight on right leg, draw left foot with loose ankle close to right foot, not touching floor. Then move left foot to west, straightening knee, and place left foot parallel to right foot. Body is on slant to northeast. While moving leg, move left arm in a downward curve, in toward body waist high; then move it up to northwest. Look at left palm as arm moves up to northwest. Do not tilt head downward. Head moves from right to left sides. (Figure 12)

Pivoting on left heel, turn left toes toward the northwest, at the same time bending left knee to equal that of right knee. Weight is equal on both legs. Back is straight and torso faces *north.* While you move left toes, turn left hand to face northwest. You are now looking at back of left hand. Legs, arm, eyes, and head, finish together. You are facing north. (Figure 100)

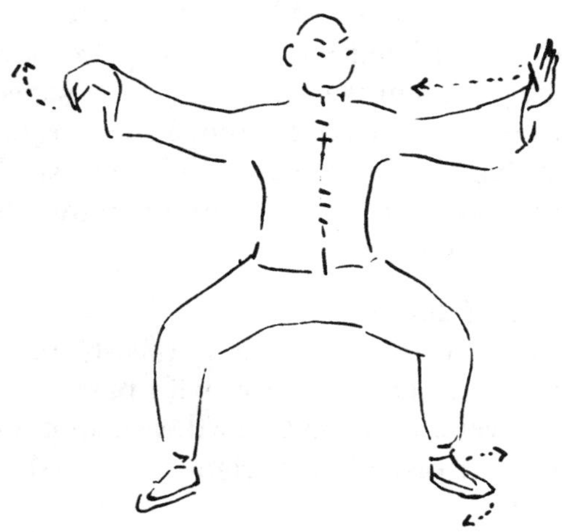

Figure 100

SERIES IV

Form 61. Hand Strums the Lute SHOU HUI P'I-P'A

Keep weight on left leg with its bent knee. Move toes of left foot inward to point northeast and then move left heel outward to west, straightening right knee. At the same time, torso is being turned to face northeast. As you move left toes and heel, both arms move: bending left elbow down, bring hand in toward left shoulder and begin to lift right hand upward. Torso faces northeast. (Figure 101)

Keeping weight on left leg with its bent knee, raise right toes up, flexing right foot. At the same time, torso is turned to east. With leg and torso movement, move left hand forward east and place left fingers at right pulse, palm facing inward. Right palm faces east, with fingers pointing to ceiling. Right foot is flexed, right knee is straight, and right heel touches floor lightly. (Figure 102)

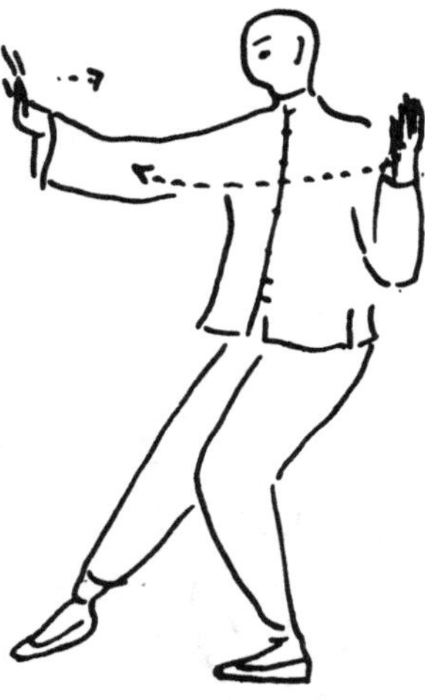

Figure 101

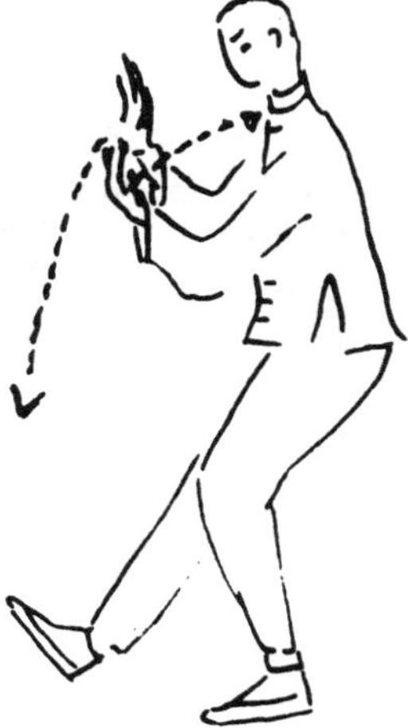

Figure 102

Form 62. Parting the Wild Horse's Mane YEH MA FEN TSUNG
On right side

Do not move feet. Bend more deeply on left knee and at the same time lean torso from hips diagonally forward and down, keeping back straight. At the same time, both arms move: place left palm in front of right shoulder, with elbow pointing downward. Straightening right arm, bring it diagonally downward across body, so that left elbow and right inner elbow meet. This movement pulls shoulders forward but not up. Right palm faces northwest, with fingers pointing toward floor to northeast. Wrists are straight. (Figure 103)

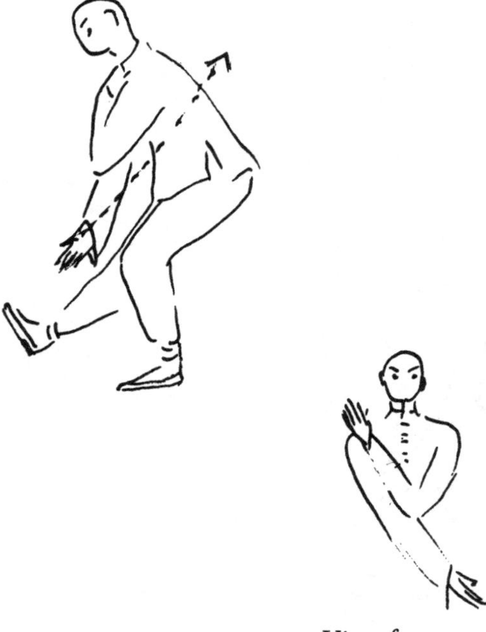

View from eas'

Figure 103

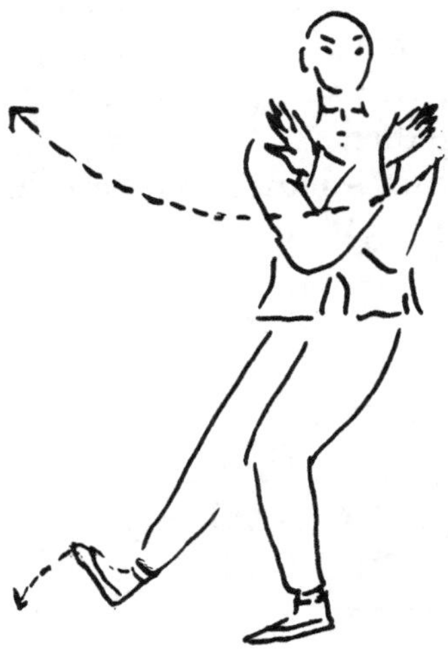

Figure 104

Keep weight on left leg with its bent knee, and do not move right flexed foot. Lift torso up and turn it to face north: hips are even and torso does not slant. At the same time, both arms move: bend right arm upward, keeping elbow even with left elbow. Face right palm in front of left shoulder and turn left palm outward to face north, keeping hand in front of right shoulder. Arms are crossed at middle of forearms; right arm is on outside; elbows are down and apart. (Figure 104)

Place weight on right leg, bending right knee and straightening left knee. At the same time body and both arms move: slant body toward east, keeping head and torso facing north. Move right arm forward north at shoulder level, with palm up; continue to move it in a horizontal circle toward east where it stops above shoulder level, in line with right shoulder, palm up. Turn left palm to east and, bending wrist, move arm downward and stop hand waist high in space between body and right arm. Head faces north. Legs, arms, and body move together.

Then, as a separate movement, turn head to east and look at right palm. (Figure 105)

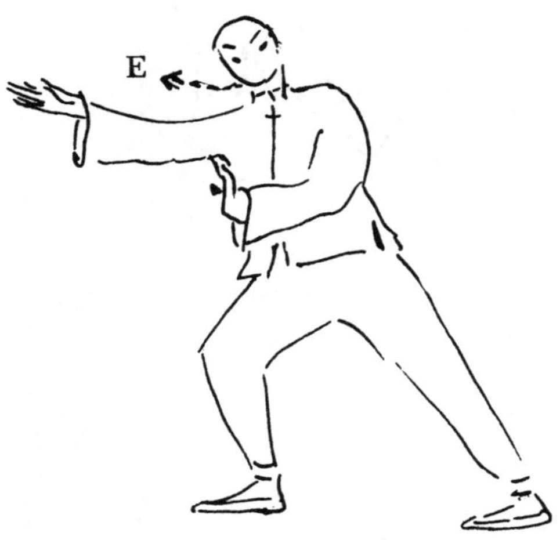

Figure 105

Form 63. Hand Strums the Lute SHOU HUI P'I-P'A

Same as Form 61, Figure 102

Turning torso to face east, shift weight back onto left leg, bending its knee, straightening right knee, and flexing right foot. At the same time, both arms move: turn right palm to face east bending elbow downward, and place left fingers at right pulse, palm facing inward. (Figure 102)

Form 64. Parting the Wild Horse's Mane YEH MA FEN TSUNG

On right side—same as Form 62, Figures 103, 104, 105.

Do not move feet. Bend more deeply on left knee and at the same time lean torso from hips, diagonally forward and down; keep back straight. At the same time both arms move: place left palm in front of right shoulder, with elbow pointing downward. Straightening right arm, bring it diagonally downward across body, so that left elbow and right inner elbow meet. This movement pulls shoulders forward. Right palm faces northwest with fingers pointing toward floor to northeast; wrists are straight. (Figure 103)

Keep weight on left with its bent knee and do not move right flexed foot. Lift torso up and turn it to face north: hips are even and torso does not slant. At the same time, both arms move: bend right arm upward, keeping elbow even with left elbow. Face right palm in front of left shoulder, and turn left palm to face north, keeping hand in front of right shoulder. Arms are crossed at middle of forearms; elbows are down and apart. (Figure 104)

Place weight on right leg, bending right knee and straightening left knee. At the same time body and both arms move: slant body toward east and keeping head and torso north. Move right arm forward north with palm up; continue to move it in a horizontal circle toward the east where the arm stops above shoulder level in line with right shoulder. Palm is up. Turn left palm to east, and bending wrist, move arm downward and stop hand waist high in the space between body and right arm. Head faces north. (Figure 105)

Then, as a separate movement, turn head to east and look at right palm.

Parting the Wild Horse's Mane
On left side

Turn head so that you are looking south: do *not* move rest of body. (Figure 106)

Keep weight on right leg, with slant of body diagonally to east. Turn torso to face east; head remains looking south as Figure 106 above. At the same time as torso moves, place right palm in front of left shoulder, bending elbow downward. Straightening left arm, bring it diagonally downward across body so that right elbow and left inner elbow meet. Left palm faces southwest, with fingers pointing toward floor to southeast. Wrists are straight. The direction of torso is east; head is south; weight is forward on right leg. (Figure 107)

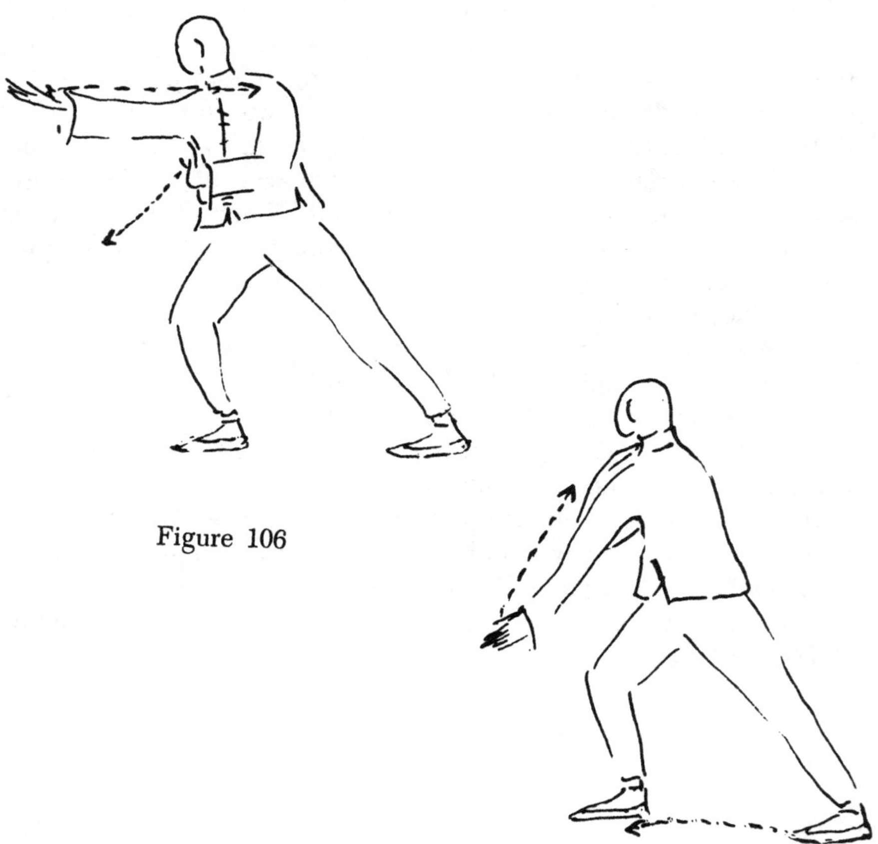

Figure 106

Figure 107

Draw left foot close to right foot, not touching floor. At the same time, cross arms and turn torso to south. Bend left arm upward, keeping elbow even with right elbow. Face left palm in front of right shoulder, and turn right palm outward to face south, keeping hand in front of left shoulder. Arms are crossed at middle of forearms, left arm is on the outside, and elbows are down and apart. (Figure 108)

Place left heel forward east in the Walking Step Space; transfer weight onto left leg, bending its knee and straightening right knee. Head remains looking south; torso faces south, and body slants forward east. At the same time, both arms move: move left arm to south at shoulder level, with palm up, and continue to move it in a horizontal circle toward east where arm stops above shoulder level in line with left shoulder. Palm is up. Turn right palm east and bending wrist, move hand downward and stop hand waist high in space between body and left arm. Legs, arms, and body move and finish at the same time. Head is facing south. (Figure 109)

Then, as a separate movement, turn head to east and look at left palm.

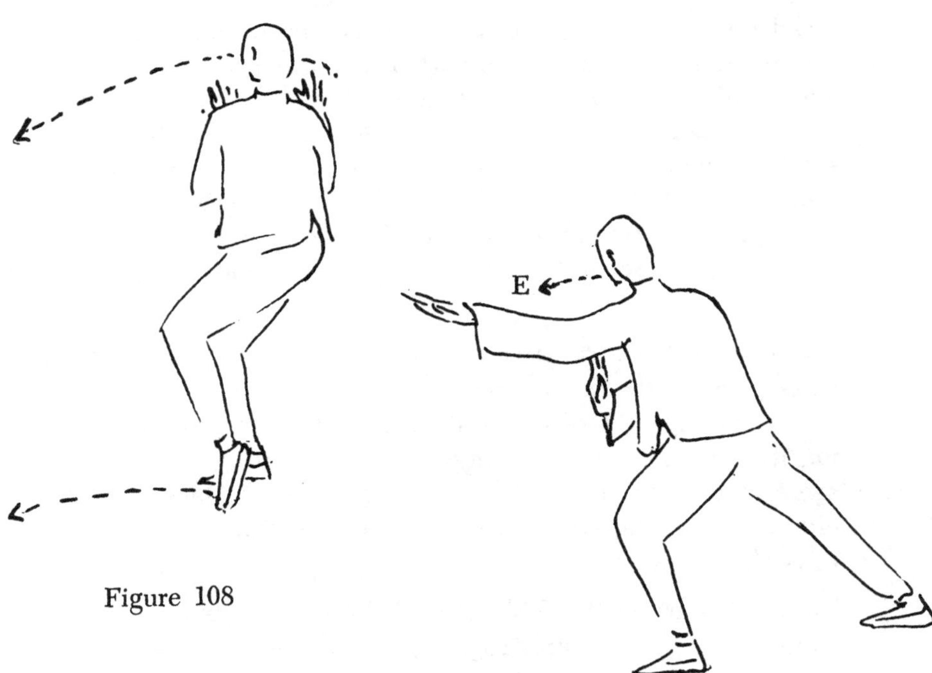

Figure 108

Figure 109

Parting the Wild Horse's Mane
On right side—same as Form 62, Figures 104, 105

Turn head so that you are looking north; do not move body. (Figure 110) Keep weight on left leg, with diagonal slant of body to east. Turn torso to face east, head remains looking north. At the same time as torso moves, place left palm in front of right shoulder, bending elbow downward. Straightening right arm, bring it diagonally downward across body so that left elbow and right inner elbow meet. Right palm faces northwest with fingers pointing toward floor to northeast. Wrists are straight.

Draw right foot close to left foot, not touching floor. At the same time, cross arms and turn torso to face north: bend right arm upward, keeping elbow even with left elbow. Face right palm in front of left shoulder, and turn left palm to face north keeping hand in front of right shoulder. Arms are crossed at middle of forearms; right arm is on the outside; elbows are down and apart. Right leg, arms, and torso move and finish positions at the same time. (Reverse of Figure 108)

Place right foot forward east in the Walking Step Space; transfer weight onto right leg, bending its knee and straightening left knee. Head remains looking north, torso faces north, and body slants to east. At the same time move both arms: move right arm forward to north with palm up; continue to move it in a horizontal circle toward the east where the arm stops above shoulder level in line with right shoulder. Palm is up. Turn left palm east, and bending wrist, move arm downward and stop hand waist high in the space between body and right arm. Head faces north. (Figure 105)

Then, as a separate movement, turn head east and look at right palm.

Form 65. Hand Strums the Lute SHOU HUI P'I-P'A
Same as Form 63, Figure 102

Turn torso to face east and shift weight back onto left leg bending its knee, straightening right knee and flexing right foot. At the same time, both arms move; turn right palm to face east, bending elbow downward, and place left fingers at right pulse, palm facing inward. (Figure 102)

Form 66. Parting the Wild Horse's Mane YEH MA FEN TSUNG
Same as Form 62, Figures 103, 104, 105. Do not omit (see page 122).

Do not move feet. Bend more deeply on left knee and at the

same time lean torso from hips diagonally forward and down. Keep back straight. At the same time both arms move: place left palm in front of right shoulder with elbow pointing downward. Straighten right arm bring it diagonally downward across body, so that left elbow and right inner elbow meet. Right palm faces northwest, with fingers pointing toward floor to northeast. Wrists are straight. (Figure 103)

Keep weight on left with its bent knee and do not move right flexed foot. Lift torso up and turn it to face north: hips are even and torso does not slant. At the same time both arms move: bend right arm upward, keeping elbow even with left elbow. Face right palm in front of left shoulder and turn left palm to face north, keeping hand in front of right shoulder. (Figure 104)

Place weight on right leg, bending its knee and straightening left knee. Move arms and body at the same time: slant torso east and keep torso and head facing north. Move right arm forward north with palm up; continue to move it in a horizontal circle toward the east where the arm stops above shoulder level in line with right shoulder. Palm is up. Turn left palm to east and bending wrist, move arm downward, stopping hand waist high between body and right arm. Head faces north. (Figure 105)

Then, as a separate movement, turn head to east and look at right palm.

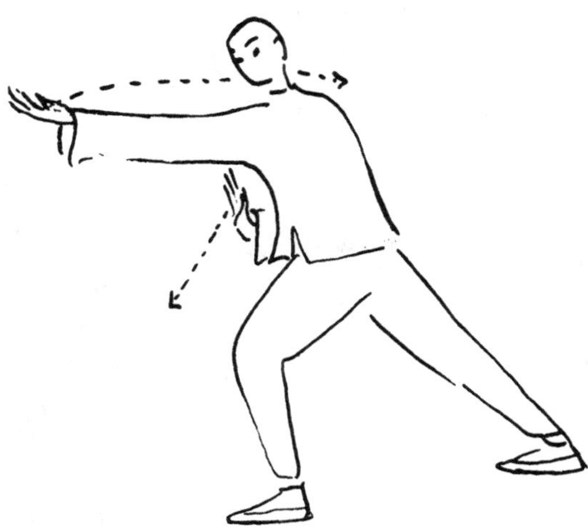

Figure 110

Form 67. Jade Girl (Angel) Works at the Shuttle

YÜ NÜ CH'ÜAN SO

On left side facing east

Keep weight on right leg. Draw left foot with loose ankle close to right foot not touching floor, and turn torso to east. At the same time both arms move: place right palm above left shoulder with elbow shoulder high, and lower left arm, placing it in front of body abdomen high, with palm facing floor and fingers pointing south. Left arm is curved with elbow pointing north. (Figure 111)

Place left heel forward east in the Walking Step space; transfer weight onto left leg, bending its knee and straightening right knee. Body slants east. At the same time move arms: raise left curved arm up east (elbow points north) so that arm is at chin level: palm faces east. Bend wrist sideways up, making hand slant upward slightly. Move right hand near left forearm with palm facing east, and place right fingertips two inches from left wrist: right wrist is bent and elbow points down. In this relationship, right finger-tips are at mouth level. (Figure 112)

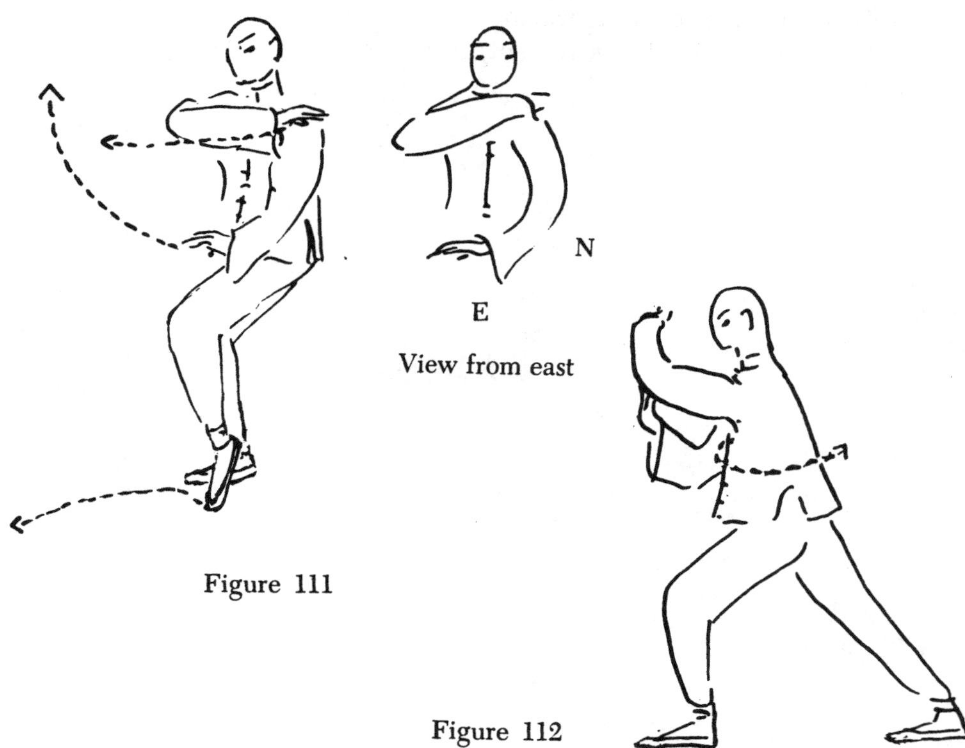

Figure 111

Figure 112

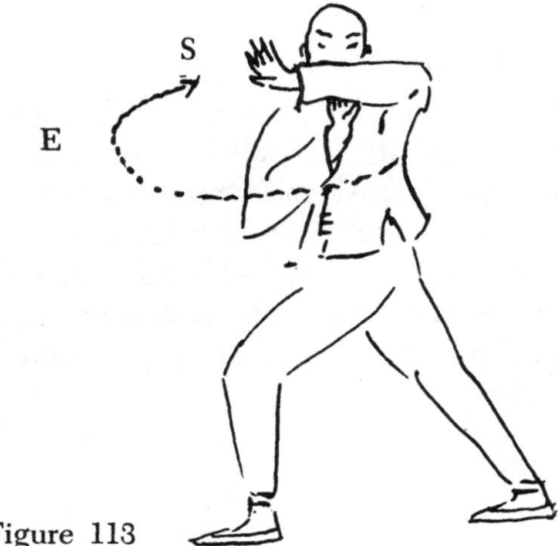

Figure 113

Keep body on a slant. Do not move legs. Keeping arms and head in same relationship to body, twist at waist and move upper torso to face north. (Figure 113)

Then move torso to east.

Now move torso to south. (Figure 114)

Again move torso back to east. During this waist-circling movement do not change level of head. (Figure 112)

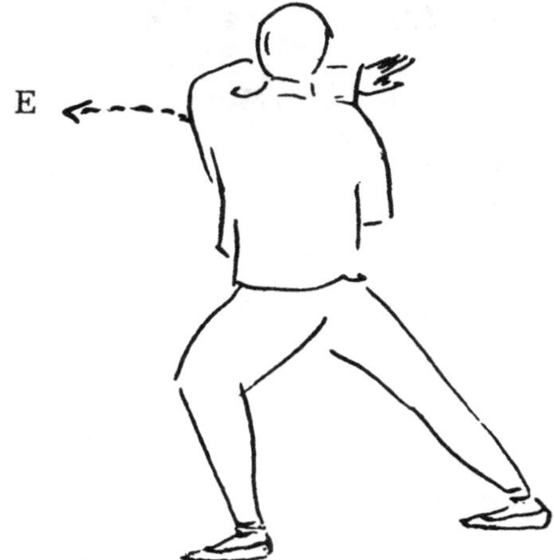

Figure 114

Form 68. Jade Girl (Angel) Works at the Shuttle

YÜ NÜ CH'ÜAN SO

On right side facing west

Keeping weight on left leg, turn toes of left foot to south; turn right heel inward making foot parallel to left with weight on left; next turn left heel out to east and straighten right knee; then flex right foot. While you do this Toe-Heel-Heel step and are turning torso to face west, both arms move: place left palm above right shoulder with elbow shoulder high, and lower right arm curved downward with palm facing floor, placing it in front of body, abdomen high. (Figure 115)

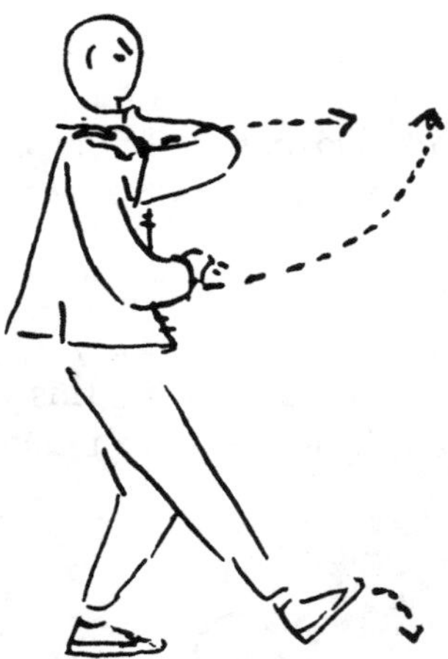

Figure 115

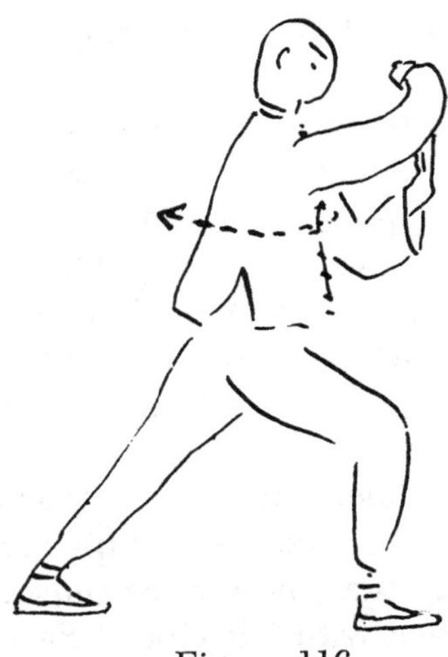

Figure 116

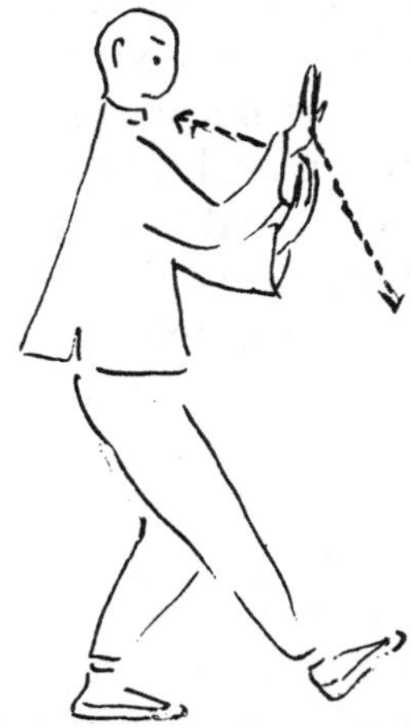

Figure 117

Place right heel forward west in the Walking Step Space; transfer weight onto right leg, bending its knee and straightening left knee. Body slants forward west. At the same time both arms move: raise right arm curved up west so that arm is at chin level; palm faces west and wrist bends sideways-up, making hand slant upward slightly. Move left hand near right forearm with palm facing west, and place fingertips two inches from right wrist; left wrist is bent and elbow points down. (Figure 116)

Do not move legs. Keep body on a slant. Keeping arms and head in same relationship to body, twist at waist and move upper torso to face north.

Then move torso to face west.

Then move torso to face south.

Now move torso back to west. During this waist-circling movement do not change level of head. (Figure 116)

Form 69. Hand Strums the Lute SHOU HUI P'I-P'A

Same as Form 63, except that here you face *west*

Shift weight back onto left leg, bending its knee and straightening right knee, and flexing foot. At the same time, both arms move: move right arm a bit inward bending elbow downward; keep palm facing west, with fingers pointing upward. Place left fingers at right pulse, facing left palm inward. (Figure 117)

Form 70. Parting the Wild Horse's Mane YEH MA FEN TSUNG

On right side—same as Form 62, Figures 103, 104, 105, except that here you face west

Do not move legs. Bend more deeply on left knee and at the same time, lean torso from hips, forward and diagonally down. Keep back straight. At the same time arms move: place left palm in front of right shoulder, with elbow pointing downward. Straightening right arm, bring it diagonally downward across body so that left elbow and right inner elbow meet. Right palm faces southeast with fingers pointing toward floor to southwest. Wrists are straight. (Figure 103)

Keep weight on left leg with its bent knee, and do not move right flexed foot. Lift torso up and turn it to face south; hips are even and torso does not slant. At the same time, both arms move: bend right arm upward, keeping elbow even with left elbow. Face right palm in front of left shoulder and turn left palm outward to face south; elbows are down and apart. (Figure 104)

Place weight on right leg, bending right knee and straightening left knee. Slant body toward west, and keep torso and head facing south. Move right arm to south and continue to move it in a horizontal circle toward west where arm stops above shoulder height in line with right shoulder. Palm is up. Turn left palm west, and bending wrist, move arm downward and stop hand waist high in space between body and right arm. Head faces south. Legs, body, and both arms all move together. (Figure 105)

Then, as a separate movement, turn head to west and look at right palm.

Form 71. Jade Girl (Angel) Works at the Shuttle

YÜ NÜ CH'ÜAN SO

Left side, facing west, Figures 111, 112, 113, 114

Keep weight on right leg. Draw left foot with loose ankle to right foot not touching floor, and turn torso west. At the same time both arms move: place right palm above left shoulder with elbow shoulder high and lower left arm, placing it in front of body abdomen high, palm facing floor, with fingers pointing north. Left elbow points south. (Figure 111)

Place left heel forward west, in the Walking Step Space; transfer weight onto left leg, bending knee and straightening right knee. Body is on a slant west. At the same time, both arms move: raise left curved arm up west (elbow is south) so that arm is at chin level:

palm faces west, and wrist bends sideways-up, making hand slant upward slightly. Move right hand near left forearm and place fingertips two inches from left wrist; right palm faces west; wrist is bent, and elbow points down. (Figure 112, except that here you face to west)-as in Figure 118.

Keep body on a slant. Do not move legs, keeping arms and head in same relationship to body; twist at waist and move upper torso to face south.

Then move torso to face west.

Then move torso to north.

Now move torso to west. During this waist-circling movement do not change level of head. (Figure 118)

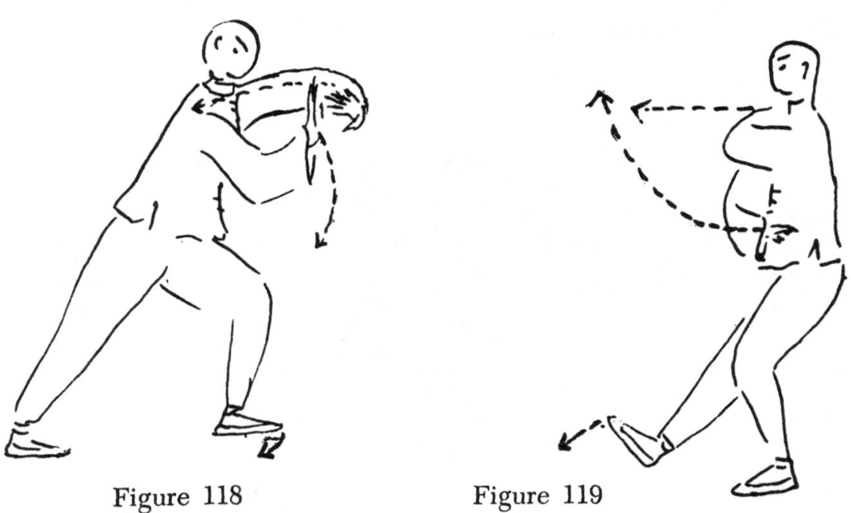

Figure 118 Figure 119

Form 72. Jade Girl (Angel) Works at the Shuttle

YÜ NÜ CH'ÜAN SO

On right side, but this time you face east

Keep weight on left leg. Turn toes of left to point north; move right heel inward making foot parallel to left foot; turn left heel outward to west and straighten right knee; then flex right foot. While you do this Toe-Heel-Heel step, and are turning torso to east, both arms move: place left palm above right shoulder with elbow shoulder high and lower right curved arm downward with palm facing floor, body abdomen high. (Figure 119)

Place right heel forward to east in the Walking Step Space; transfer weight onto right, bending its knee and straightening left knee. Body is on a slant to east. Both arms move at the same time as leg moves: raise curved right arm up to east at chin level, point elbow south, and face palm to east. Wrist bends sideways-up so that hand is slanted upward slightly. Move left hand near right forearm and place finger tips two inches from right wrist. Palm faces east. Left wrist is bent and elbow points down.

Do not move legs. Keep body on a slant. Keeping arms and head in same relationship to body, twist at waist and move upper torso to face south.

Then move torso to face east.

Then move torso to face north.

Then move torso to face east. (Figure 120) During this waist-circling movement, do not change level of head.

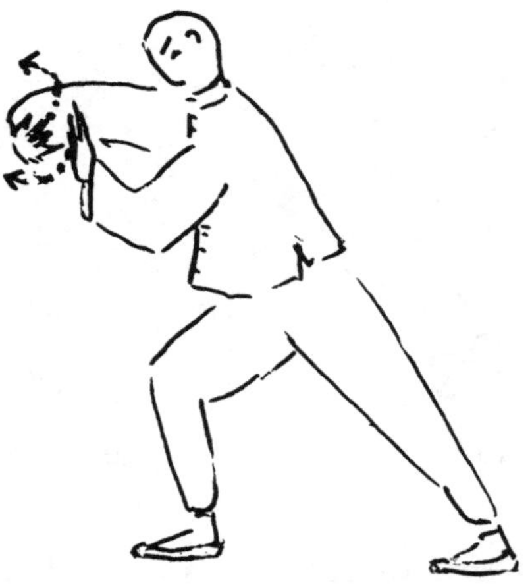

Figure 120

Form 73. Hand Strums the Lute SHOU HUI P'I-P'A
Facing east, same as Form 63, Figure 102

Shift weight back onto left leg, bending knee, straightening right knee and flexing foot. At the same time, both arms move: move right arm bending elbow downward, keeping palm east with right fingers pointing upward. Place left fingers at right pulse with left palm facing inward. (Figure 102)

Form 74. Parting the Wild Horse's Mane YEH MA FEN TSUNG
On right side, Form 62, Figures 103, 104, 105

Do not move feet. Bend more deeply on left knee and at the same time lean torso diagonally forward and down. At the same time both arms move: place left palm in front of right shoulder with elbow pointing downward. Straightening right arm, bring it diagonally across body so that left elbow and right inner elbow meet. Right palm faces northwest with fingers pointing toward floor to northeast. Wrists are straight. (Figure 103)

Keep weight on left leg with its bent knee, and do not move right flexed foot. Lift torso up and turn it to face north. At the same time, both arms move: bend right arm upward and place palm in front of left shoulder, and turn left palm outward to face north, keeping hand in front of right shoulder. Arms are crossed at middle of forearms, the right on the outside, with elbows down and apart.

Place weight on right foot, bending right knee and straightening left knee. At the same time body and both arms move: slant body to east, keeping torso and head facing north. Move right arm north at shoulder level with palm up; continue to move it in a horizontal circle toward east where arm stops above shoulder level in line with right shoulder. Turn left palm to east, and bending wrist, move arm downward and stop hand waist high in space between right arm and body. Head faces north. Leg, body, and arms move together. (Figure 105)

Then, as a separate movement, turn head to east and look at right palm.

Form 75. Grasping the Bird's Tail LAN CH'ÜEH WEI
Same as Forms 2, 3, 4, Figures 7, 8, 9, 10, 11

Shift weight back onto left leg, bending its knee, straightening right knee, and flexing foot. At the same time, move both arms: placing left finger tips at right pulse, keep right fingers pointing east, turning right palm to face north, and turn left palm to face south: both elbows are curved downward. Hands are at face level. (Figure 7)

Keeping the relationship of hands the same, move both arms inward toward body at chin level, bending both elbows downward and slightly out. Do not come too close to face.

Turn right palm up and left palm down at the same time. As you move hands, angle left hand so that it is at right angles to right wrist, so that left elbow points north. (Figure 8)

Step on right foot, bending its knee and straightening left knee. Body is on slant forward east. At the same time, stretch right arm to northeast, straightening right elbow. Left fingers remain at right pulse. Arms are chin level high. (Figure 9)

Circle both arms horizontally, chin high, from northeast, to east, to south, to southwest. When arms reach south, bend right elbow downward and bend right wrist so that palm faces upward. With right fingers leading the movement, both left and right fingers point southwest at the end of this horizontal circling. Left arm is adjusted to movement of the right, because left fingers always remain near right pulse. (Figure 10)

As you are circling arms from south to southwest, shift weight back onto left leg, bending its knee, straightening right knee, and flexing right foot. (Figure 10)

Pivot on right heel, turning toes to northeast, and place foot on floor. At the same time, raise right arm with palm leading up toward ceiling, circle it over and down toward northeast, straightening right arm as you do so, and stop in position where right wrist is slightly above shoulder height. (Figure 11)

As you are approaching this last arm position, bend right knee, placing weight on right leg and straightening left knee. At the same time, bend right wrist and lower hand making fingers point downward in Grasping position. Right arm remains in place while hand moves. Left fingers remain near right pulse, with palm facing you. (Figure 11)

Form 76. The Single Whip TAN PIEN

Same as Form 5, Figures 12 and 13

Hold weight on right leg with its bent knee. Draw left foot with loose ankle close to right one, not touching floor. Then move left leg backward to southwest diagonal in the Walking Step Space. Straighten left knee and place foot parallel to right foot. Weight is on right leg; body is on a slant to northeast. As left leg moves, move left arm with palm toward face in a downward curve, circling in toward body waist high. Left arm is curved and palm is toward your face. Right arm does not move. (Figure 12)

Pivoting on left heel, turn toes toward the northwest. Place weight on left leg and bend left knee to equal that of right knee. Now your weight is even on both legs. Body is turned to northwest. Feet are separated by a distance equal to twice the length of your foot. Your back is straight.

As left foot moves, turn left palm to face the northwest. Now both arms are on the same level, with wrists higher than shoulder level. (Figure 13)

Keep looking at left palm as hand moves to northwest. Move head from right to left sides. Do not bend head when eyes look downward. When left palm turns to northwest, you will then be looking at the back of left hand.

Synchronize movements of eyes, arm, legs, head, and body. (Figures 12 and 13)

Form 77. Cloud Arms YÜN SHOU

Same as Form 32, Figures 62, 63, 64, 65, 66. Do not omit (see page 13).

Do not move right arm. Turn left toes inward to point north and then move left heel outward to make foot parallel to right foot. With the movements of left foot, shift weight onto right leg and straighten left knee: body slants to northeast. At the same time as you move left foot and shift weight, circle left arm downward and then inward to body, waist high, keeping wrist bent. Gradually straightening wrist, move left arm upwards toward right wrist. Place left fingers near right pulse, with palm inward facing you. As left arm moves, raise right hand slowly upward, opening hand to face palm northeast. Left foot, left arm, and right hand move together. (Figure 62)

Shift weight back onto left leg, bending left knee and straightening right knee. At the same time, both arms move: looking at left palm, move left arm to left side with palm at eye level, twelve inches away from face. Keep eyes fixed on palm. At the same time, circle right arm outward to right side, and then downward, with bent wrist and palm facing down. (Figure 63)

Keeping weight on left leg, turn right toes inward to point northwest. Then turn left toes outward to point northwest. As feet move, torso moves to face northwest. Along with feet and torso, both arms move: continue to move left arm, face high, to left side, with eyes looking at palm. Continue to move right arm in its circle from downward to inward waist high in front of body, gradually straightening wrist. Then move hand upward toward left hand. (Figure 64)

Keeping weight on left leg, place right foot parallel and apart from left in your basic stance: both toes point northwest; both knees are evenly bent; back is straight; torso faces northwest. Both arms continue to move: turn left palm to face northwest, at eye level, while you move right fingers up to left pulse, turning right palm to face your face. Look at right palm now. Both elbows point downwards. (Figure 65)

Turn torso toward right to face northeast and move right arm to right side, with palm at eye level, twelve inches away from face. Eyes look at right palm. Then turn right toes to point northeast, placing weight onto right leg with its bent knee. Then turn left knee inward, touching left toes to floor with loose ankle, thus taking weight off left foot. At the same time as right arm and torso turn to northeast, move left arm: circle left arm with wrist bent and palm down, outward to left side and then downward. Continue to circle it inward to body waist high, gradually straightening wrist. Then move it up toward the right pulse. (Figure 66)

As left hand goes upward toward right side, place left leg diagonally backward to southwest in the Walking Step Space. Straighten left knee and bend right knee more deeply with weight on right leg. Body slants to northeast. On this last movement, turn right palm out to face northeast, and place left fingers at right pulse with palm toward face. Eyes look far away to northeast while left hand, right hand, left foot, and shifting eye gaze are made simultaneously. (Figure 62)

Repeat all of Cloud Arms from Figure 62. Go to 63, 64, 65, 66, and 62 again in exactly the same way. Do not omit this repeat (See page 13).

Form 78. The Single Whip **TAN PIEN**

Same as Form 5, Figures 12 and 13

Continue this from the repeat of Figure 62. Bend right wrist downward and place fingers down in Grasping position. Then move left arm downward, and inward toward waist. (Figure 12)

Continue left arm upward, northwest. Turn left palm to face northwest and turn left toes also to northwest; bend left knee to equal that of right knee. Back is straight. As left arm moves, look at palm as it moves downward and upward. Move head from right to left side. Look at back of left hand on its last movement. Torso faces northwest. (Figure 13)

SERIES V

Form 79. The Snake Creeps Down SHE SHEN HSIA SHIH

Do not move head. Turn left toes slightly inward, and at the same time turn left palm inward facing east. Then shift weight onto left leg, straightening right knee; at the same time, bend both hands so that palms face upward and fingers point west. As right hand turns upward, move right arm west toward left hand and above head: hands are fifteen inches apart. (Figure 121)

With palms facing ceiling, move both hands, with fingers leading, in a horizontal circle from west, to south, to northeast; fingers finish pointing to northeast. As hands move from west, weight is on left leg, with right knee straightened and right toes touching floor. As arms move from south to northeast, step out on right foot and shift weight onto right leg, bending its knee and straightening left knee. (Figure 122)

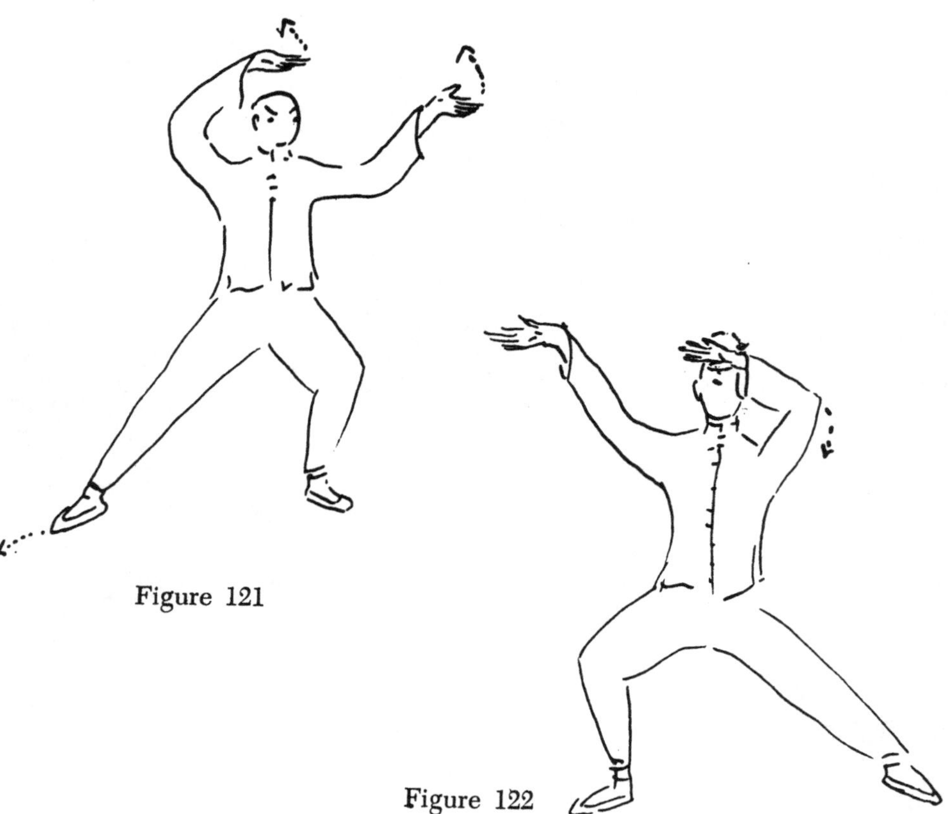

Figure 121

Figure 122

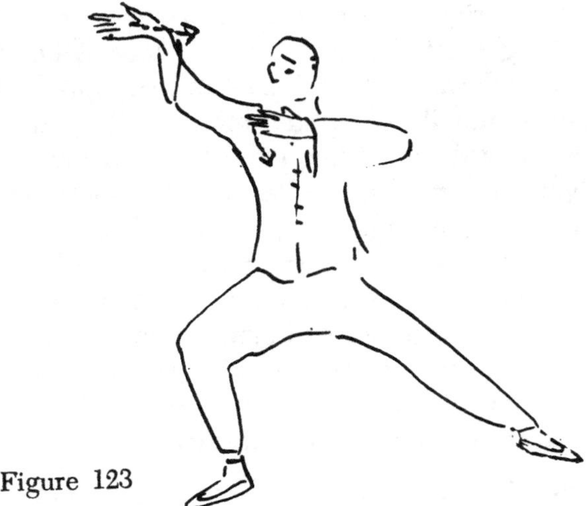

Figure 123

Keep weight on right leg. Turn left palm inward to face your face, lowering arm at the same time. Then bend right wrist so that palm faces inward with fingers pointing to left hand; right arm stays high; right and left hands and arms are on a diagonal. (Figure 123)

Bend left wrist so that hand is turned back: in this position left palm faces right fingers and left fingers point north. Keep right elbow high. As left hand moves, lower left elbow. (Figures 122, 123, and 124 move consecutively.) With these hand movements both arms also move: move arms downward toward left foot, on a diagonal line from high point at right northeast to low point above left foot at southwest. (Figure 124)

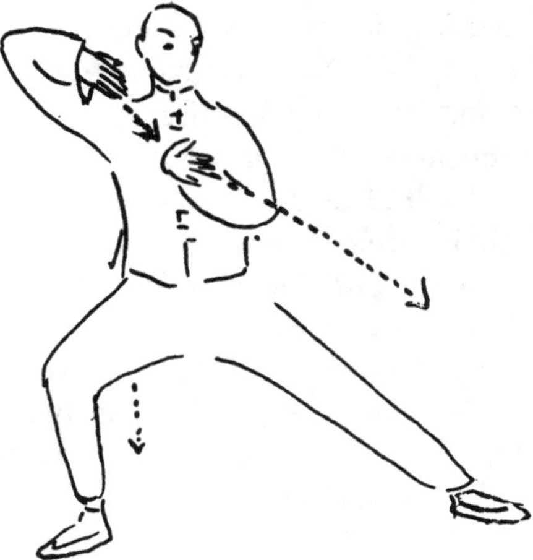

Figure 124

Lower body on right side by bending right knee more deeply. Keep left leg straight. At the same time as knee is bending, both arms continue their downward diagonal movement. Move left elbow to left side, and gradually straighten elbow and straighten wrist: left arm finishes on a diagonal line parallel to left leg. At the same time, move right arm, with fingers leading, in exactly the line the left arm is making: right fingertips point to left palm; right elbow stays high and bent. Finish right arm movement with straightened wrist, when right fingertips are near left inner elbow. Both arms complete their movements together and simultaneously, with the deep knee bend on right leg. As arms are moving in their diagonal line down toward left leg, turn torso slightly toward left. Arms move close to body. Head remains looking northwest. (Figure 125)

Form 80. Golden Cockerel Stands on One Leg CHIN CHI TU LI
Right side

Shift weight onto left leg, bending its knee. At the same time, both arms move: start to raise left arm up to left with fingers to west, and move right arm vertically downward with fingers pointing to floor. Wrists are straight. (Figure 126)

At the same time as arms move, turn right toes to point west, straightening right knee. Then move left heel inward to make foot parallel with right: weight is on left leg with its bent knee. The movements of right toes and left heel turn torso to face west. Body is on a slant forward west. While you shift toes and heel, complete the movements of arms. Move left arm upward in line with left shoulder, with palm north and fingers west; and move right arm downward vertically at right side, with palm inward toward body and fingers pointing downward. (Figure 127)

Weight is on the left: draw right foot with loose ankle to left foot not touching floor. Then raise it up high toward west: right knee is high and lower part of leg is held high, with flexed foot. At the same time, both arms move: move right arm toward west, then upward and then circle it inward toward forehead. Turn back of hand to forehead: palm faces west, elbow is curved and points north. Move left arm in a curve inward toward chest, and then outward to meet right knee: place hand with palm west above right knee: elbow points south. Right leg and both arms move and finish movements together. Left knee is slightly bent. Torso is slightly curved forward. (Figure 128)

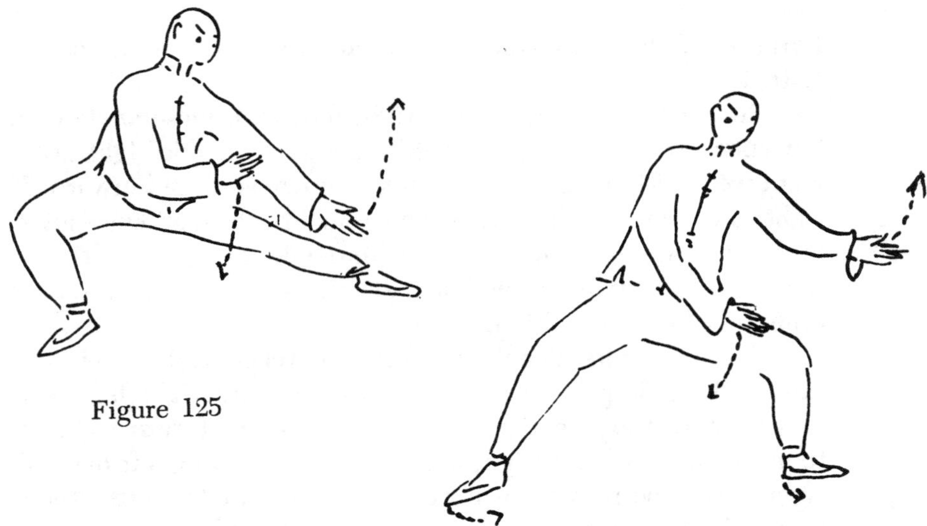

Figure 125

Figure 126

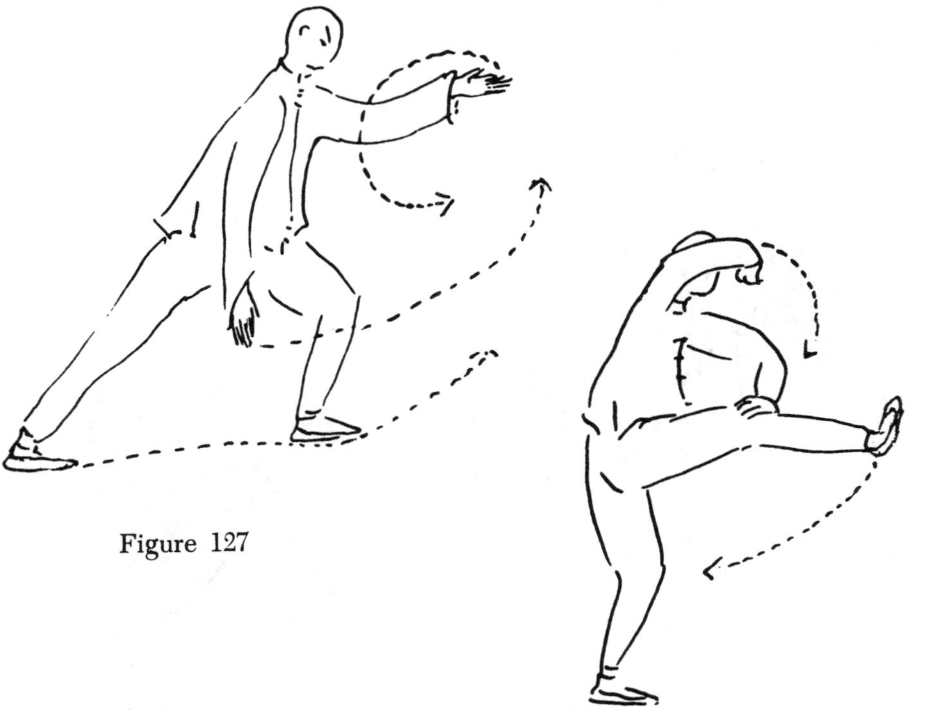

Figure 127

Figure 128

Form 81. Golden Cockerel Stands on One Leg CHIN CHI TU LI
Left side

Bend right knee and bring right foot with loose ankle close to left knee. At the same time, both arms move: circle right arm outward west with palm out, and circle it downward and inward. Place right hand under left hand which remains at right knee level. At the same time as right palm goes under it, turn left palm to face upward. Right palm faces knee. Backs of hands are toward each other, not touching. (Figure 129)

Bending more deeply on left leg, reach right heel west in the Walking Step Space. Transfer weight onto right leg, bending its knee and straightening left knee. Body slants forward west. Start to move hands when weight is on right leg. Keeping left hand above right, circle both arms in a vertical circle out to north, then upward. (Figure 130)

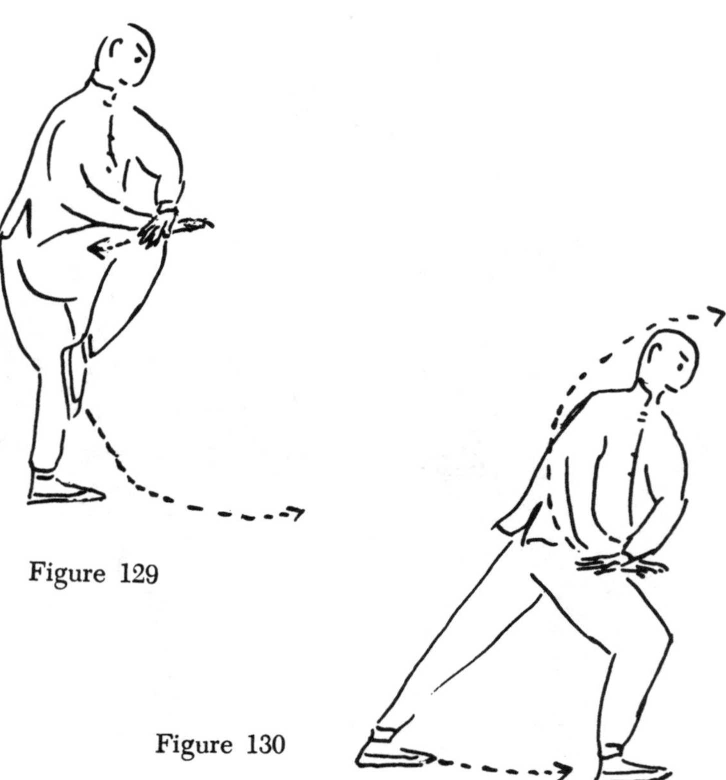

Figure 129

Figure 130

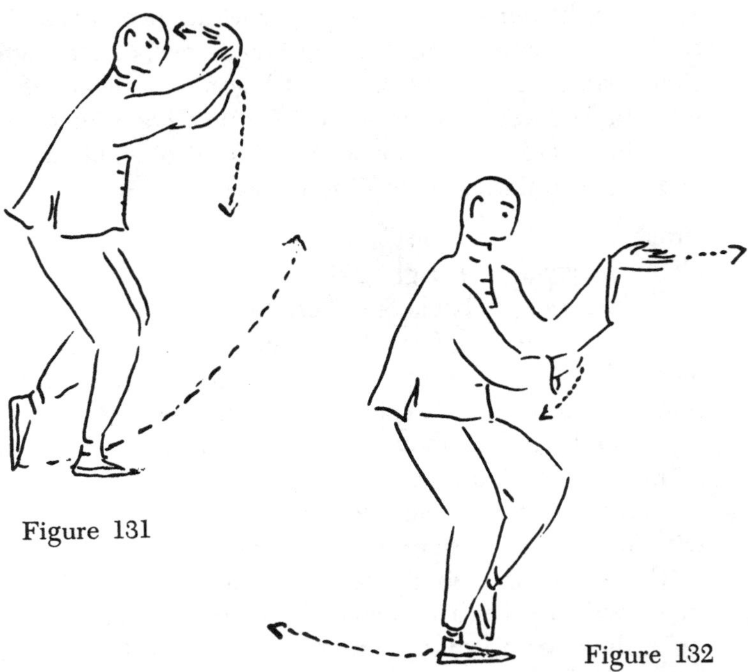

Figure 131

Figure 132

Continue to move arms high inward toward forehead. As you do so, draw left foot with loose ankle over to right foot, and start to raise it up toward west. (Figure 131)

Separate hands: circle right arm downward and place right hand above left knee with palm west. At the same time, turn left hand, which is already at forehead, to face palm west. Left leg is now up high to west, knee is bent, and lower leg is high, with foot flexed. (Opposite of Figure 128)

Form 82. Brush Knee Twist Step LOU HSI NIU PU

Backward on left side, same as Form 20, Figures 47, 48, 49, 25.

Bring left elbow down and bend wrist so that fingers point west with palm north: wrist is at shoulder level. At the same time, bend left knee and move left foot with loose ankle to right knee, and bend more deeply on right knee. Keep right hand above right knee. (Figure 132)

Lower left foot with loose ankle close to right foot, not touching floor. Gradually move right arm to right. (Figure 47)

Weight remains on right leg with its bent knee. Place left foot backward to east in the Walking Step Space, and straighten its knee; Body slants forward west. As left leg moves, move left arm forward west in line with left shoulder, turning hand to face west; while right hand finishes its movement at front of right thigh, palm down and fingers pointing west. (Figure 48)

Brush Knee Twist Step
Going backward on right side

Shift weight back onto left leg, bending its knee; straighten right knee, and flex foot. Move left hand inward to center twelve inches from chest, keeping elbow high: palm is west with fingers pointing north. At the same time as leg and left hand move, move right hand upward above left wrist, with fingers pointing west and palm south. (Figure 49)

Keep weight on left leg with its bent knee. Draw right foot with loose ankle close to left. Then place right foot backward to east in the Walking Step Space, straightening right leg. At the same time, both arms move: move right arm forward west in line with right shoulder, turning palm to west. Circle left arm downward to front of left thigh with palm down and fingers pointing west. (Figure 25)

Brush Knee Twist Step
Going backward on left side

Shift weight back onto right leg bending its knee, straighten left knee, and flex foot. Draw right hand inward toward center, twelve inches from chest, keeping elbow high: palm faces west and fingers point south. At the same time, move left hand upward above right wrist, with fingers pointing west and palm facing north.

Keep weight on right leg. Without touching floor, draw left foot with loose ankle to right foot. Place left leg backward to east in the Walking Step Space, straightening left knee. Body slants forward west. At the same time, both arms move: move left arm forward west in line with left shoulder, turning palm west, and circle right arm downward to front of right thigh, with palm down and fingers pointing west. (Figure 48)

Form 83. Flying Oblique HSIEH FEI SHIH

Same as Form 21, Figures 50, 51, 52, 53

Keep weight on right leg with its bent knee. Foot, hand, and head move together. Turn toes of right foot to northwest. Turn right palm up, keeping fingers pointing west. Bend head down, and turn chin toward right shoulder. Do not move arms or shoulders; do not shift weight from right leg. Movements are made in ankle, wrist, and neck. (Figure 50)

Keep weight on right leg with its bent knee. Draw left foot with loose ankle inward to right foot, not touching floor. Bend more deeply on right knee, bending torso slightly downward. At the same time, circle right fingers inward to body, keeping palm up. (Figure 51)

Move left foot outward toward southwest as far as it can go with a straight knee. Place left foot parallel to right foot, so that both feet point northwest. At the same time continue to circle right hand with palm up inward to northeast: fingers point to northeast. (Figure 52)

Shift weight onto left leg, bending its knee, and straighten right knee. Bend torso forward and sit as low as you can on left leg: body faces northwest; head looks toward northeast. At the same time as body lowers over onto left side, turn left palm up with fingers pointing west and straighten wrist. At the same time, turn right palm down with fingers pointing to northeast. Right arm is parallel to right leg. Look at back of right hand. All movements finish together. (Figure 53)

Form 84. Raise Hands and Step Up T'I SHOU SHANG SHIH

Same as Form 6, Figures 16, 17, 18

Turn right toes to point north and shift weight onto right leg, bending its knee and straightening left knee. On these movements, keep body low; torso turns to face north. Then turn toes of left foot to point north. At the same time as legs move, both arms move: bring right arm in a curve forward and shoulder high, fifteen inches from body. Move left hand with palm turned to northeast toward inner curve of right elbow. Left elbow points downward and right elbow is shoulder high. (Figure 16)

Draw left foot up to right and place it parallel and apart from right foot in your basic stance. Both knees are equally bent and torso is curved forward north. At the same time, arms complete the movements described above: right is curved forward shoulder high and left palm is at inner curve of right elbow. (Figure 17)

Raise body to an upright position, at the same time straightening knees. Also at the same time, lift curved right arm to a position above forehead, and lower left arm, with palm down, to front of left thigh; wrist is bent and fingers point north. Arms, body, and legs finish together. (Figure 18)

Then as a separate movement, turn right hand to face palm upward.

Form 85. White Stork Flaps Its Wings PAI HAO LIANG CH'IH

Same as Form 7, Figures 19, 20, 21, 22, 23

Do not move right arm from its place above forehead for the next sequences.

Bend torso forward down, and at the same time, move left arm away from thigh so that it is perpendicular to floor. Palm faces floor. (Figure 19)

Keep arms in same relative positions. Twist torso around to west, keeping body low. Arms move with body. Now left fingers point west. (Figure 20)

Lift torso up erect, remaining turned toward west. At the same time bring straight left arm up to shoulder height. Left wrist is bent with palm west and fingers point upward. Head and torso are turned west; knees are straight. (Figure 21)

Turn torso to north. As you do this, bend left elbow and bring left hand to center of forehead with palm north so that left fingers point to right fingers. (Figure 22)

Bend both knees, keeping back straight. At the same time, move both hands: bend wrists and turn hands so that palms face diagonally downward front. At the same time as hands move, press elbows diagonally forward so that right elbow points northeast and left elbow points northwest, both being at shoulder level. Make this movement with strength and hardness. Feel the contraction in the muscles of upper arms. This contrasts with the light and soft movement you have been using up to now. Feel as if you were holding or pressing a huge ball between elbows and hands. Knees and hands move together (Figure 23)

Form 86. Brush Knee Twist Step LOU HSI NIU PU

Same as Form 8, Figures 24, 25

Keep weight on right leg with its bent knee. Shift right heel to east. This movement turns torso to face west, and at the same time, weight is released from left leg. Then straighten left knee and flex foot. As you move body and legs to west, turn right palm inward toward forehead, and turn left palm outward. Then circle left arm outward and downward, and move right arm down to shoulder level. Continue to circle left hand under right hand as right hand circles above left wrist. By this time, you are facing west. Both hands are twelve inches away from chest: right palm faces south with fingers pointing west. Left wrist is bent with fingers north and palm west. (Figure 24)

Moving left heel to west, place left heel in the Walking Step Space, with straight knee and flexed foot. Then transfer weight onto left leg, bending its knee and straightening right knee. Body slants forward west. As you step west, both arms move: move right arm to west in line with right shoulder, turning palm to face west with fingers pointing upward. At the same time, circle left arm with bent wrist downward and place left hand at front of left thigh. Palm faces floor with fingers pointing west. (Figure 25)

Form 87. Hand Strums the Lute SHOU HUI P'I-P'A

Same as Form 9, Figure 26

Shift weight back onto right leg bending right knee, and at the same time straighten left knee and flex foot. As legs move, both arms move: bring right arm inward twelve inches from face, keeping palm facing west with fingers pointing up. Move left hand upward and place fingertips at right pulse: left palm faces toward heart. Arms and legs move at the same time. (Figure 26)

Form 88. Needle at the Bottom of the Sea HAI TI CHEN

Same as Form 26, Figure 54

Draw left foot, with loose ankle, to right foot, touching toes lightly on floor. Weight is on right leg. At the same time, lower torso by bending more deeply on right knee and lean torso forward on a diagonal. Keep spine straight—do not curve back. On body and leg movement, start to move both arms: turning right palm south and left palm north, move right arm diagonally downward, with straight wrist, and gradually straighten right elbow. At the same time, move left palm close along right forearm to right inner elbow: left wrist bends gradually. Right arm is straight; left wrist and elbow are bent. Arms, legs, and body finish movements together. (Figure 54)

Form 89. Fan Through the Back SHAN T'UNG PAI
Same as Form 27, Figures 55, 56, 57

Keep weight on right leg. Raise torso and direct it to northwest angle. At the same time, lift both arms, pointing right fingers up to northwest angle, at shoulder level. Right fingers point northwest and left hand remains at right inner elbow.

Then place left foot in front of right, with its heel in line with right toes, turning left toes inward to point northwest. Straighten left knee. Right knee is close to left leg. Head looks northwest. (Figure 55)

Shift weight onto left leg, bending left knee and straightening right knee. At the same time, begin to move both arms: slide (without touching) left fingers along right forearm toward northwest and draw right arm to right side. Left fingertips are at right palm when left knee is bent and right knee is straight. (Figure 56)

Keeping weight on left bent leg, move right heel slightly inward, making foot parallel to left. Then turn right toes outward to point northeast, bending right knee to equal that of left knee bend. You are now seated evenly on both legs, facing northeast. As you move right heel and toes, continue to move both arms: move left arm, which is shoulder high, to northwest with palm facing northwest and fingers up, and move curved right arm forehead high, to right side of head. Then turn right palm outward and up when arm gets into position. Left arm is straight, right arm is curved. Eyes look at back of left hand. (Figure 57)

Form 90. Turn Body—Throw Fist FAN SHEN P'IEH SHEN CH'UI
Same as Form 28, Figures 58, 59

Keeping weight on left leg with bent knee, move left toes inward to northeast. Then move left heel outward to west, and on this heel movement straighten right knee. Keep right foot on floor. As left toes and heel move, upper torso is shifted to face northeast; head remains looking north. While you move left toes and heel, both arms move: circle left arm downward, making hand into a fist, and place it near left hipbone, with fist-palm facing down. Circle right arm, gradually making hand into a fist, outward to east, then downward and inward to left hip. Place right fist above left with fist-palm down. Both fists arrive in position at the same time with movements of left toes and heel. When fists meet, pull shoulders forward, moving elbows slightly forward. Use a hard force similar to Pressing the Ball. (Figure 58)

Move right toes to point east, shifting weight onto right leg, bending its knee, and straightening left knee. Body slants forward east. At the same time, both arms move: move right fist up to east, chin high, with fist-palm facing east; wrist is bent. Move left fist, gradually opening hand and spreading fingers wide apart, and place behind right fist. Wrist is bent: left palm is behind right fist, with left fingers pointing upward. Both elbows are low. (Figure 59)

Form 91. Step Up, Parry, and Punch CHIN PU PAN LAN CH'UI

Shift weight back onto left leg bending knee, straightening right knee and flexing foot. At the same time, both hands move: turn left palm to face south and gradually place fingers together. Turn right fist to face left palm. Draw right fist along left forearm (not touching it) and start to draw it back toward right hip, turning right fist-palm upward, elbow moving back to point west. Left arm remains shoulder high toward east. (Figure 133)

Shift weight forward onto right leg bending its knee, and straightening left knee. At the same time, move right fist forward east and place it in front of left palm which turns inward. (Figure 134) Draw left foot with loose ankle up to right foot.

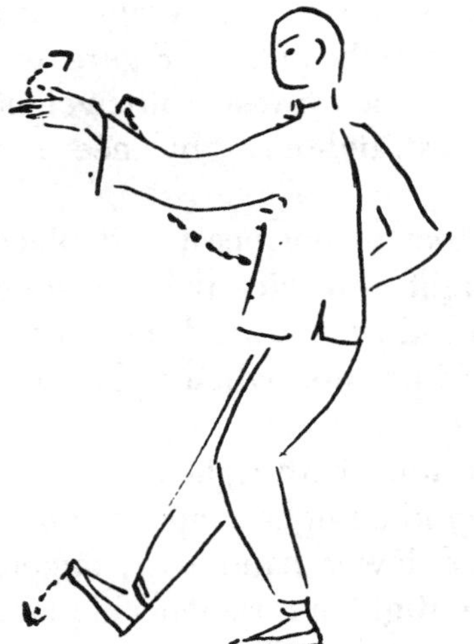

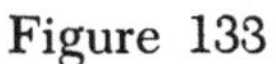

Figure 133

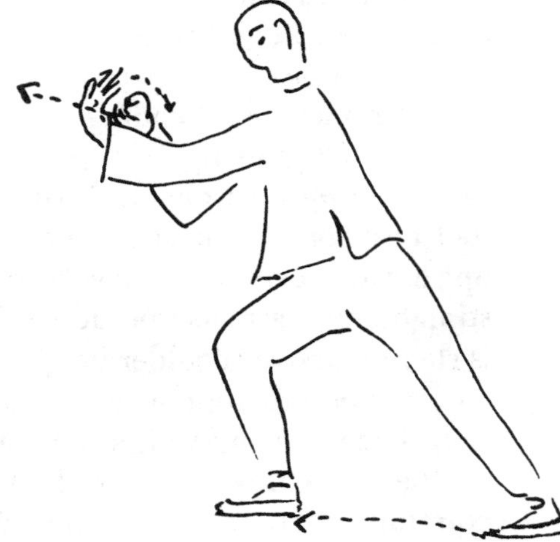

Figure 134

Form 92. Grasping the Bird's Tail LAN CH'ÜEH WEI

Same as Form 30, Figures 7, 8, 9, 10, 11

Circle left hand downward around fist (keeping close to it) and place left fingertips at right pulse. Open right hand and point fingers to east. At the same time, step forward east on left foot bending left knee and straightening right knee. Body is on a slant forward east.

Shift weight back onto right leg, bending knee, straightening left knee, and flexing foot. At the same time, draw both arms inward toward body, chin high (do not come too close), keeping hands in same relationship. Elbows bend downward. Shift weight onto left leg, bending knee and straightening right leg. Draw right foot with loose ankle close to left foot; do not touch floor. Turn right palm up and left palm down; angle left hand so that it is at right angles to right hand. (Figure 7 and Figure 8 for hands)

Then step right heel out to east in the Walking Step Space and transfer weight onto right leg, bending its knee and straightening left knee. Body is on a slant forward east. At the same time stretch right arm to northeast, straightening right elbow. Keep left fingers at right pulse. (Figure 9)

Circle both arms horizontally, chin high, from northeast to east, to south, to southwest. When arms reach south, bend right elbow downward and bend right wrist so that palm faces upward toward ceiling. Both left and right fingers point southwest at the end of this horizontal circling. Left arm is adjusted to movement of right arm because left fingertips always remain near right pulse. (Figure 10)

As you are circling arms from south to southwest, shift weight back onto left leg, bending its knee, and straighten right knee and flex foot. (Figure 10)

Pivoting on right heel, turn right toes to northeast and place foot on floor. At the same time, raise right arm with palm leading up toward ceiling. Circle it over and down toward northeast, straightening arm as you do so. Stop in a position when right wrist is slightly above shoulder height. (Figure 11)

As you are approaching this last position with right arm, bend right knee, placing weight on right leg and straightening left knee. At the same time, bend right wrist and lower hand with fingers pointing downward, in Grasping position. Right arm remains in place while hand moves. Left fingers remain at right pulse. (Figure 11)

Form 93. The Single Whip **TAN PIEN**

Same as Form 5, Figures 12, 13

Hold weight on right leg. Draw left foot with loose ankle close to right foot, not touching floor. Then move left leg to southwest diagonal in the Walking Step Space. Straighten left knee and place foot parallel to right foot. Body slants toward northeast. At the same time, move left arm down and in toward body waist high. As arm is moving, palm is toward the face. Head moves from right to left side. Eyes look at left palm as it moves. (Figure 12)

Turn left toes to point northwest. Bend left knee to equal that of right knee. Weight is even on both legs. Back is straight. Torso faces northwest. On movement of left toes, turn left hand to face northwest. Eyes look at back of left hand.

SERIES VI

Form 94. On Right—High Pat the Horse KAO T'AN MA

Same as Form 34, Figures 67, 68

Keeping weight on right leg, move right toes inward to northwest. Then move right heel outward to east and straighten left knee, keeping foot on floor. This movement on right foot turns torso to west. At the same time as you move right foot, bend right elbow downward and raise right hand upward, opening hand; and then bring hand inward toward right shoulder with palm west. Left palm now faces west. (Figure 67)

Weight remains on right leg with its bent knee. Draw left foot with loose ankle back and place it close to right foot; touch toes to floor. Back is straight. At the same time, both arms move: turning left palm upward, draw left arm inward: left elbow goes to left side at hip height. Palm is up with straight wrist. Move right arm to west with palm facing south; keep elbow high so that hand is at face level. Right elbow is bent at a right angle. Left palm is level with right elbow. Arms are separated by width of body. (Figure 68)

Form 95. Side—Face Palm P'I MIEN CHANG

Place left heel forward west in the Walking Step Space; transfer weight onto left leg bending knee and straightening right knee. Body is on a slant forward west. At the same time both arms move: place right hand with palm downward at left armpit: elbow is high. Move left arm forward west in line with left shoulder, turning palm to face west with fingers pointing upward. (Figure 135)

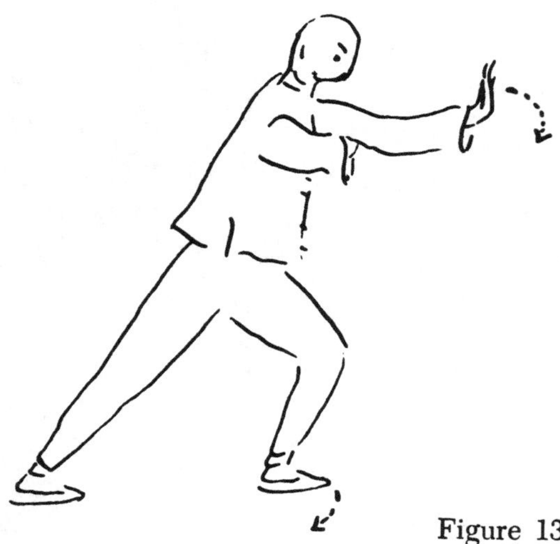

Figure 135

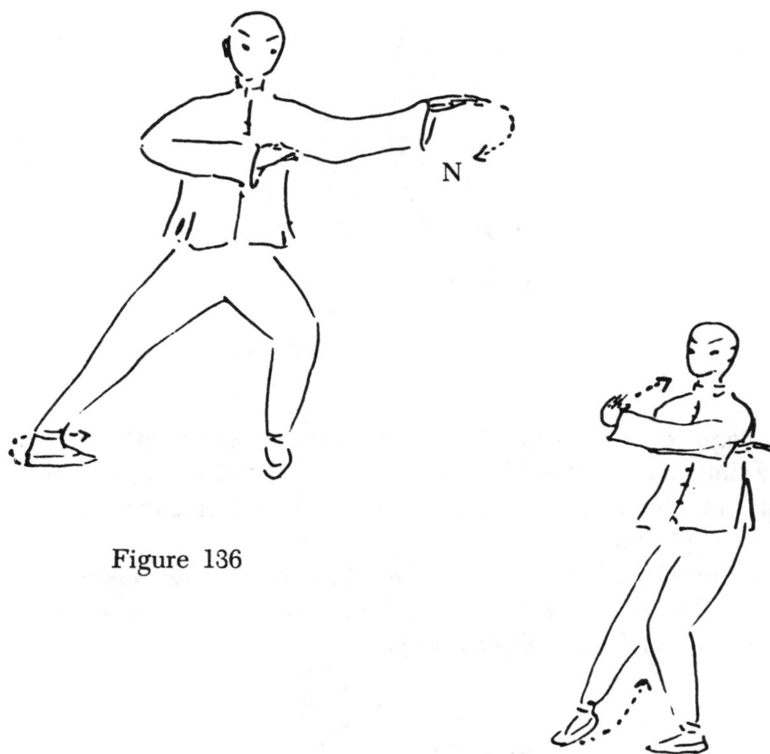

Figure 136

Figure 137

Form 96. Turn Body—Cross Leg CHUAN SHEN SHIH-TZU T'UI

Keep weight on left leg. Turn left toes inward to point north. At the same time, torso turns north and left arm moves with body: gradually straighten wrist, facing palm down, keeping shoulder high. Do not move right arm. (Figure 136)

Move right heel inward, bending right knee slightly. Then move left heel outward to west and straighten right knee; at the same time, torso and left arm move to east: move left arm at shoulder level in a horizontal circle, directing hand toward right shoulder. Do not move right arm. (Figure 137)

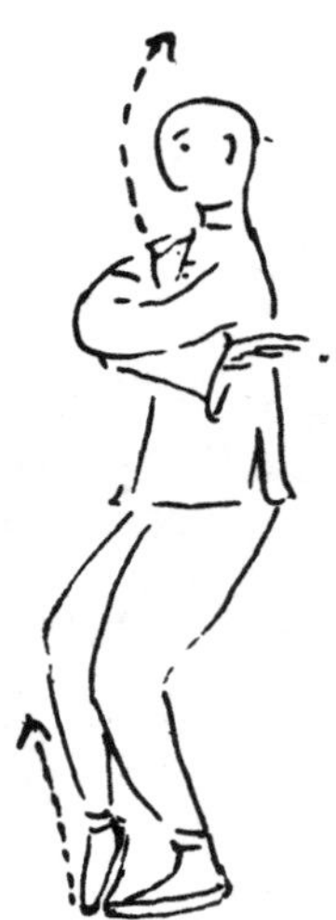

Figure 138

Begin to draw right foot with loose ankle to left foot. At the same time, left hand, with palm down and shoulder high, approaches right shoulder in its horizontal circle. Place left palm above right shoulder. (Figure 138)

Draw right knee up and place foot with loose ankle near left knee; at the same time turn left palm toward ceiling and raise curved left arm above head. (Figure 139)

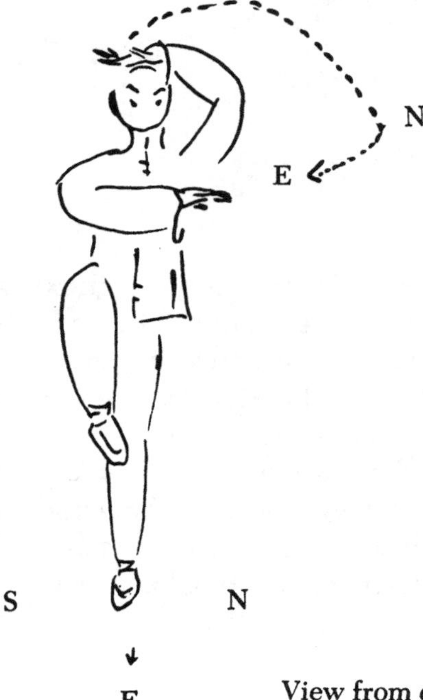

Figure 139 View from east

Continue to move left arm: move arm outward to north, shoulder high, with palm at north and fingers pointing up. Then move it in a horizontal circle at shoulder level toward east, gradually straightening wrist: palm faces down. As arm circles, extend and move right leg directly to east, with foot flexed; touch left hand to right toes. Body bends forward slightly. Extended left hand and extended right leg meet at the same time. Do not move right arm. (Figure 140)

Form 97. Straight Center Punch CHIH TANG CH'UI

Keep weight on left leg. Bend right knee and bring right leg back and place right foot with loose ankle near left knee. At the same time, draw right elbow to right hip and make a fist of right hand, pulling right elbow back to west; turn right fist-palm upward at right hip. Left arm remains at left shoulder level: turn palm south with fingers toward east, and pull left arm inward, slightly bending elbow down. (Figure 141)

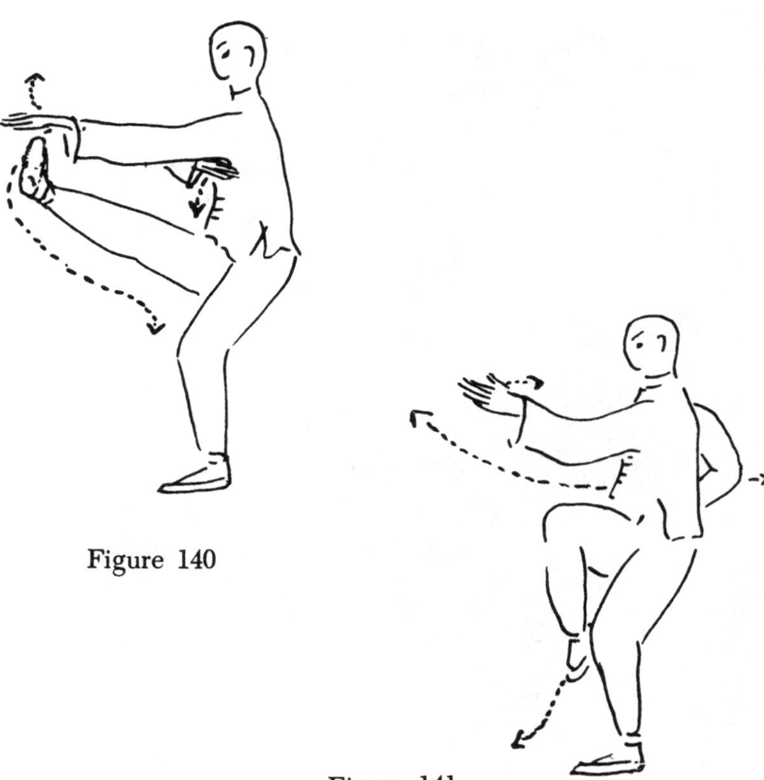

Figure 140

Figure 141

Step forward east quickly on right foot; then *quickly* step forward on left foot, bending its knee and straightening right knee. Body is on a slant forward east. This is done extremely quickly—like a flash. Move from right to left foot with a short, quick step on right. As you step quickly on right, pull right fist back at right hip and push left arm outward toward east, as if you were opening a bow to shoot an arrow.

As you step on left foot, punch right fist east, abdomen high. At the same time, move left palm to right inner elbow; wrist is bent and fingers point upward. Elbow is bent. This punch is done with hard force. Remember to keep heel of right foot on floor. (Figure 142)

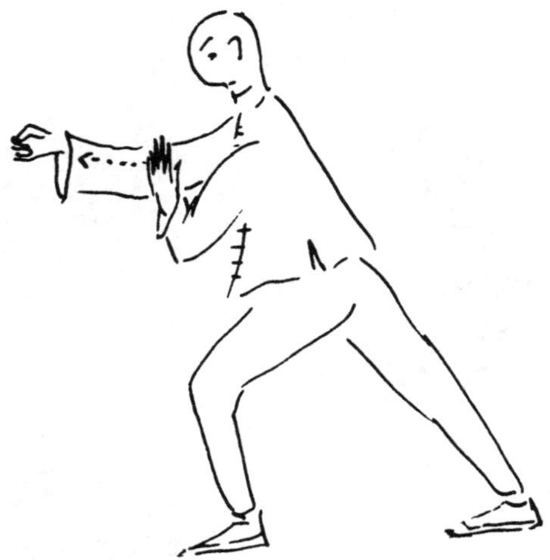

Figure 142

Form 98. Grasping the Bird's Tail LAN CH'ÜEH WEI

Same as Form 30, Figures 7, 8, 9, 10, 11

Shift weight back onto right leg, bending its knee, straightening left knee, and flexing foot. At the same time, move left fingers to right pulse and open right hand keeping fingers pointing east. (Figure 7 for arms)

Keep the relationship of hands the same: move both arms inward toward body at chin level with both elbows bent downward and slightly out. Do not come too close to body.

Turn right palm up and left palm down. As you move hands, angle left hand so that it is at right angles to right wrist: now left elbow points north. At the same time as hands turn, shift weight forward onto left leg bending its knee and straightening right knee: body is on slant forward east. (Figure 8 for arms only)

Then draw right foot with loose ankle close to left foot.

Place right heel forward east in the Walking Step space, bending right knee and straightening left knee. Body slants forward at the same time as you step forward, stretch right arm to northeast with straight elbow. Keep left fingers at right wrist. (Figure 9)

Circle both arms horizontally chin high, going from northeast, to east, to south, to southwest. When arms reach south, bend right elbow downward, bending right wrist so that palm faces upward. Both left and right fingers point southwest. Left arm is adjusted to movement of right arm. Left fingers stay at right pulse (Figure 10)

As you are circling arms from south to southwest, shift weight back onto left leg by bending left knee and straightening right knee and flexing foot. (Figure 10)

Pivoting on right heel, turn toes to northeast and place foot on floor. At the same time, raise right arm with palm leading up toward ceiling; circle it over and down toward northeast, straightening arm as you do so, and stop in position when right wrist is slightly above shoulder height. (Figure 11)

As you are approaching this last position with right arm, bend right knee, placing weight on right leg and straightening left knee. At the same time, bend right wrist and lower hand, so that fingers point downward in grasping position: right arm remains in place while right hand moves. Left fingers remain near right pulse; left palm is toward your face. Left wrist is straight and arm is curved. (Figure 11)

Form 99. The Single Whip TAN PIEN

Same as Form 5, Figures 12 and 13

Hold weight on right leg with its bent knee. Draw left foot with loose ankle close to right foot, not touching floor. Then move left leg backward to southwest diagonal in the Walking Step space. Straighten left knee and place foot parallel to right foot: weight is on right, with body on a diagonal slant toward northeast. As left leg moves, move left arm, with palm toward your face, in a downward curve, in toward body waist high. Eyes look at palm of left hand as it moves; do not tilt head. Head moves from right to left side. Right arm does not move. (Figure 12)

Continue moving left arm up and outward toward northwest, and then pivoting on left heel, turn toes to point northwest. Place weight on left leg and bend knee to equal that of right knee. Now your weight is even on both legs. Back is straight and body is turned northwest. Turn left palm to face northwest as you move left toes. Both arms are at a little above shoulder level. Head is northwest and eyes look at back of left hand. (Figure 13)

Form 100. Snake Creeps Down SHE SHEN HSIA SHIH

Same as Form 79, Figures 121, 123, 124, 125

Turn left toes slightly inward, and at the same time, turn left palm inward, facing east. Then shift weight onto left leg, straightening right knee; at the same time, bend both hands so that palms face upward and fingers point west. As right hand turns upward, move right arm to west toward left hand and above head: hands are fifteen inches apart. (Figure 121)

With palms facing ceiling, move both hands with fingers leading in a horizontal circle, from west, to south, to northeast: fingers finish pointing to northeast. As hands move from west, weight onto left leg, with right knee straightened and right toes touching floor. As arms move from south to northeast, step out on right foot and shift weight onto right leg, bending right knee and straightening left knee. (Figure 122)

Keep weight on right leg. Turn left palm inward to face your face, lowering arm at same time. Then bend right wrist so that palm faces inward with fingers pointing to left hand; right arm stays high; right and left hands and arms are on a diagonal. (Figure 123)

Bend left wrist so that hand is turned back: therefore, left palm faces right fingers and left fingers point north. Keep right elbow high. As left hand moves, lower left elbow. (Figures 122, 123, and

124 move consecutively.) With these hand movements both arms also move: move arms downward toward left foot, on a diagonal line, from the high point at right northeast, to the low point above left foot at southwest. (Figure 124)

Lower body on right side by bending right knee more deeply. Keep left leg straight. At the same time as knee is bending, both arms continue their downward diagonal movement. Move left elbow to left side and gradually straighten elbow and wrist: left arm finishes on a diagonal line parallel to left leg. At the same time, move right arm, with fingers leading, in exactly the line the left arm is making: right fingertips point to left palm; right elbow stays high and bent. Finish right arm movement with straightened wrist, when right fingertips are near left inner elbow. Both arms complete their movements together and simultaneously with the deep knee bend on right leg. As arms are moving in their diagonal line down toward left leg, bend torso slightly toward left. Arms move close to body. Head remains looking northwest. (Figure 125)

Form 101. Step Up to Form Seven Stars SHANG PU CH'I HSING

Shift weight onto left leg bending its knee. At the same time both arms move: start to raise left arm upward to left with fingers pointing to west, and move right arm vertically downward with fingers pointing to floor. Wrists are straight. (Figure 126)

At the same time as arms are moving, turn right toes to point west straightening right knee. Then move left heel inward to make foot parallel with right foot: weight is on left leg with its bent knee. The movements of right toes and left heel turn torso to face west. Body is on a slant forward west. While you shift toes and heel, complete the movements of arms: move left arm upward in line with left shoulder, with palm north and fingers west; and move right arm downward vertically at right side, with palm inward toward body and fingers pointing downward. (Figure 127)

Keep weight on left leg with its bent knee and with torso on a slant forward west. Draw right foot with loose ankle close to left foot. Then move right leg to west. Straighten knee and place foot flat on floor, toeing-in slightly. At the same time, right arm moves: bring arm up to west with palm south, and place right hand near left hand so that left thumb is at center of right palm. At the same time, when right hand reaches this position, move both wrists without moving arms out of place: bend left hand downward diagonally and spread fingers wide apart; bend right hand upward diagonally and spread fingers wide apart. (Figure 143)

Form 102. Retreat Step and Ride the Tiger T'UI PU K'UA HU

Keep weight on left leg with its bent knee. Bring right foot with loose ankle back near left foot. At the same time, both hands move: passing each other, right hand goes downward and left hand upward over right wrist. At the same time as hands are moving, draw fingers of each hand close together, so that hands are in their usual form, with palm curved and fingers close. Wrists are diagonally crossed with hands facing the diagonals: left hand faces northeast, and right hand southeast.

Keep weight on left with its bent knee. Place right leg backward to east in the Walking Step Space, straightening right knee. At the same time as leg goes back, lower torso forward down west, and bring both arms down to a perpendicular; hands are crossed at wrists. (Figure 144)

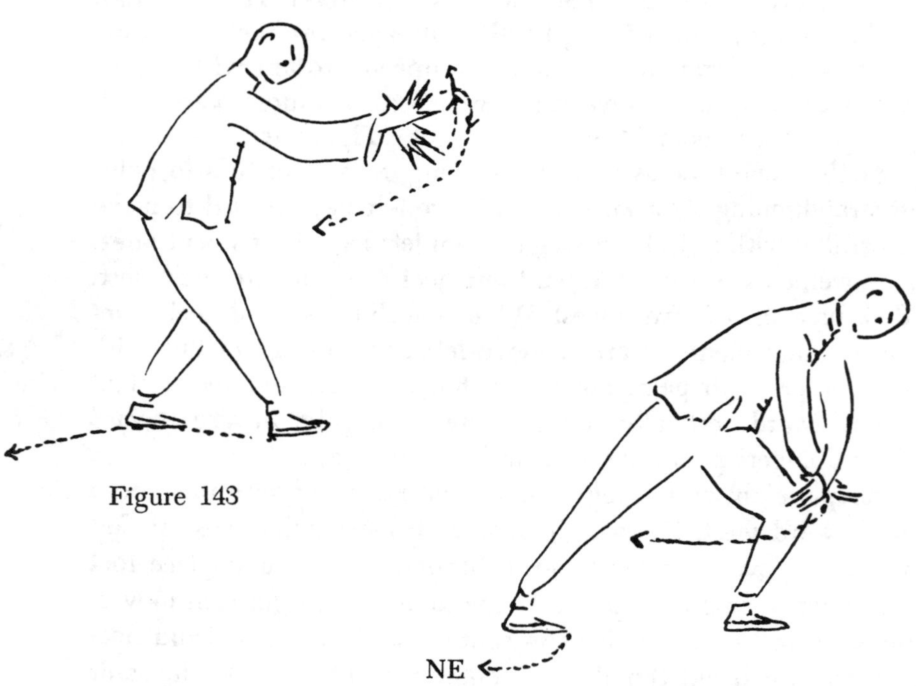

Figure 143

Figure 144

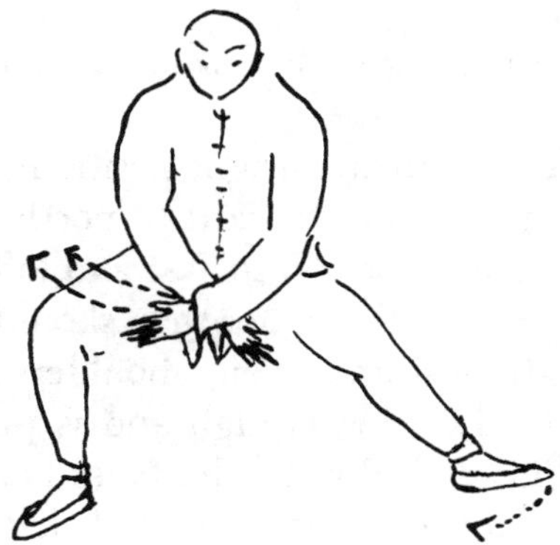

Figure 145

Move right toes to northeast and move bent-over torso to north with it, arms moving with torso; bend right knee, straightening left knee at the same time as torso moves north. Arms are now near right knee. (Figure 145)

Turn left toes to north and at the same time, bend both wrists so that fingers of both hands point east: right palm faces floor and left palm faces up. Start to fold left fingers over left thumb as wrists bend. (Figure 146)

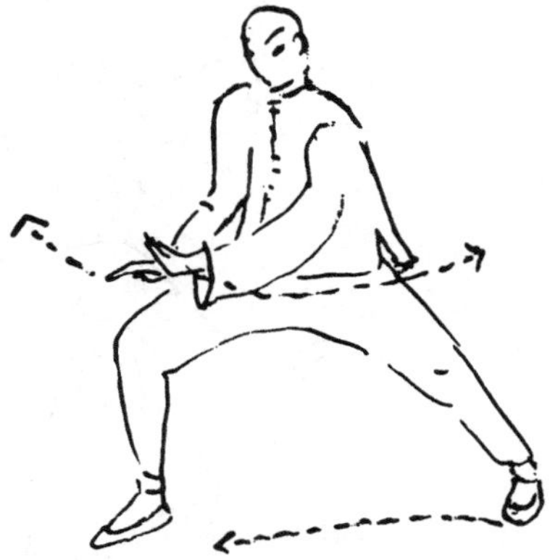

Figure 146

Separate arms at the same time: right goes up toward east with wrist bent so that fingers point upward. Left arm goes toward west with bent wrist leading and fingers pointing downward. At the same time, move left leg with loose ankle close to right foot. (Figure 147)

Begin to lift torso to an upright position; at the same time, bring left leg with bent knee up forward to northeast. At the same time, both arms move: right goes up to east and left goes up to west, until they reach positions a little higher than shoulder level. Head is front-north; hips are straight and even; shoulders are straight and even. Torso faces north. Left leg is high and is pulled over to northeast with foot flexed inward. Right palm faces northeast. Left hand is in Grasping position toward northwest. Left leg, torso, and arms arrive in position at the same time. (Figure 148)

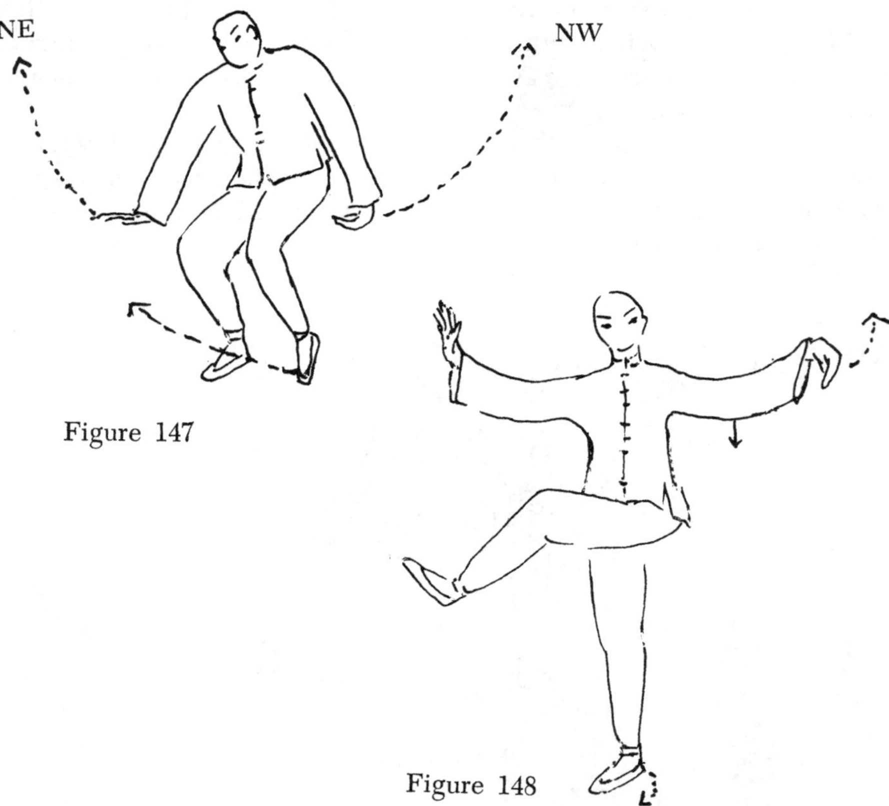

Figure 147

Figure 148

Form 103. Turn Around and Swing Leg (Lotus Swing)

CHUAN SHEN PAI LIEN

Lower left elbow downward and draw left hand toward left shoulder; at the same time, raise hand up with palm to north.

Pivot on right heel, placing toes east. This movement turns body to face east. Right arm shoulder high extends to east, palm is east. (Figure 149)

Keep weight on right leg. Bend more deeply on right knee, lowering body, and place left foot on floor to east with toes inward and with straight knee. At the same time, place right hand with palm down at left armpit and extend left arm to east in line with left shoulder: palm is east. (Figure 150)

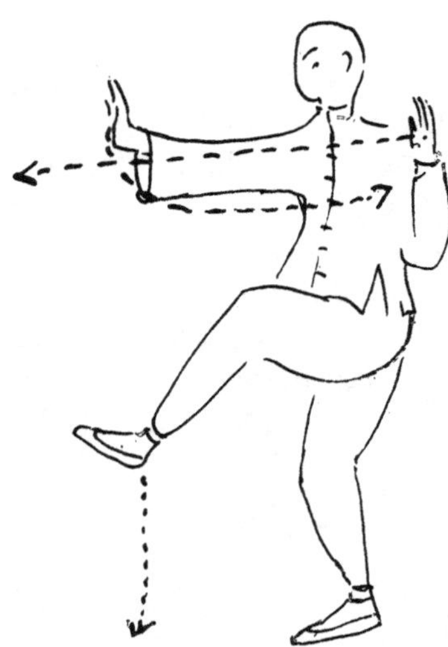

Figure 149

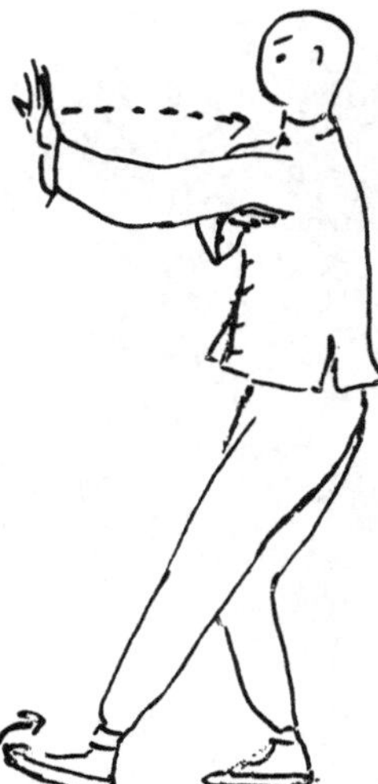

Figure 150

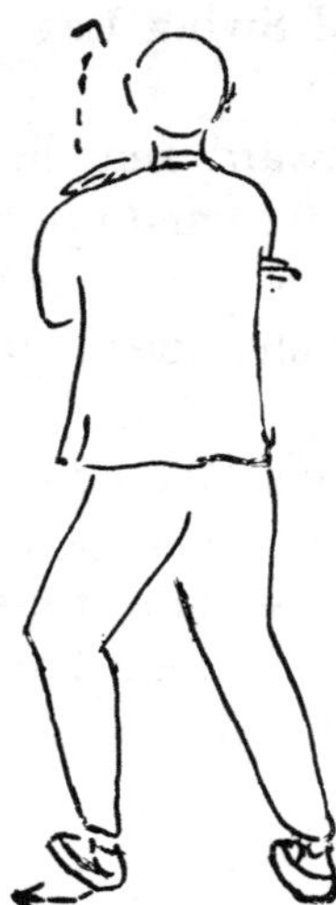

Figure 151

Turn left toes inward to south and shift weight onto left leg, bending its knee and straightening right knee. Then move right heel inward and bend knee slightly. At the same time, place left hand with palm down, at right armpit, and place right hand above left shoulder. Elbows are shoulder high. (Figure 151)

Continue with the Toe-Heel-Heel step. Moving left heel outward to east, raise right arm curved above head, with palm up. Torso now faces west. Left arm does not move. (Figure 152)

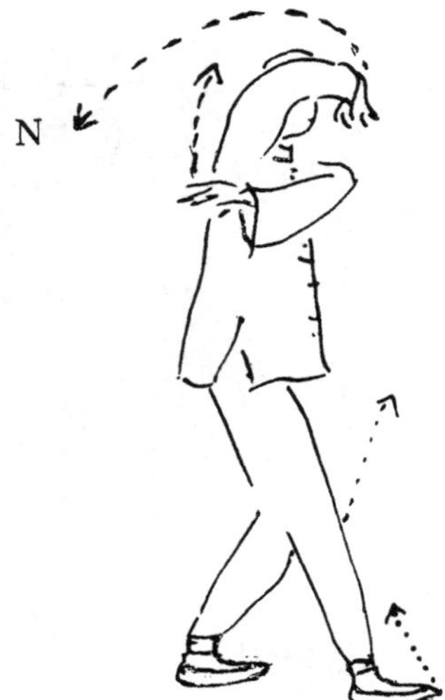

Figure 152

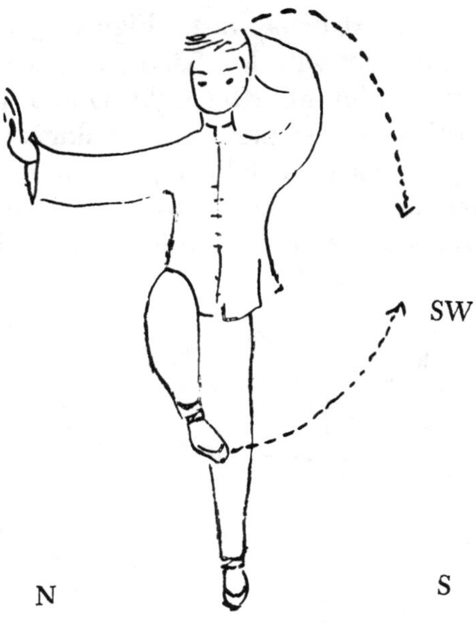

Figure 153. View facing west

Lift right leg and bring foot with loose ankle near left knee: right knee points west and right foot is toed in. At the same time as leg lifts, both arms move: move right arm out to north shoulder high with palm facing north and fingers up. Move left arm up curved, above head, with palm up. (Figure 153)

Swing-circle right leg very *quickly:* swing it to southwest and then to west. (Figure 154, A and B)

Quickly place foot down in the Walking Step Space west. Body slants forward west. (Figure 155)

For Figure 154 arms must move quickly: (a) slap-strike right foot on its inner side with left palm as foot swings to southwest. (b) Slap-strike right foot on its outer side with right palm as right foot swings to west. Bend body down and toward west in order to strike foot. The tempo is extremely fast. (Figure 154, A and B)

After striking foot with left hand, bring arm up curved in front of forehead, with palm up. After right hand strikes, bring right arm up toward northwest with palm up and fingers pointing northwest. The arms go into place as right leg goes into Walking Step Space with bent knee: left knee straightens. Hands are about twelve inches apart. Left arm is curved and right is straight. (Figure 155)

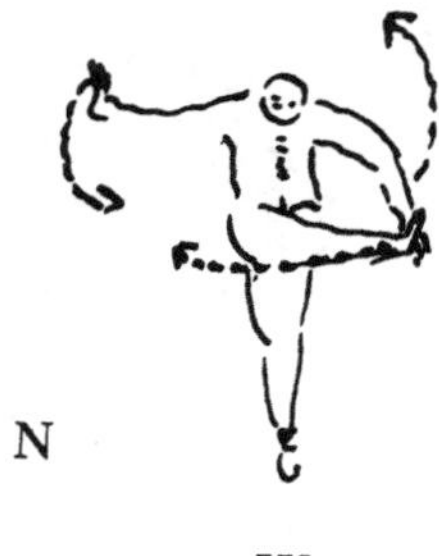

View facing west

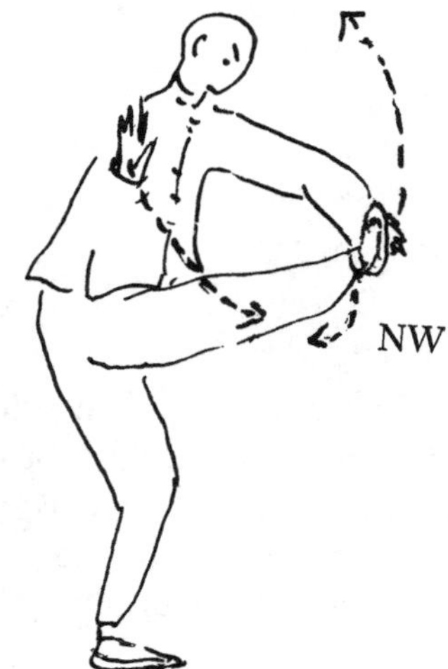

Figure 154A

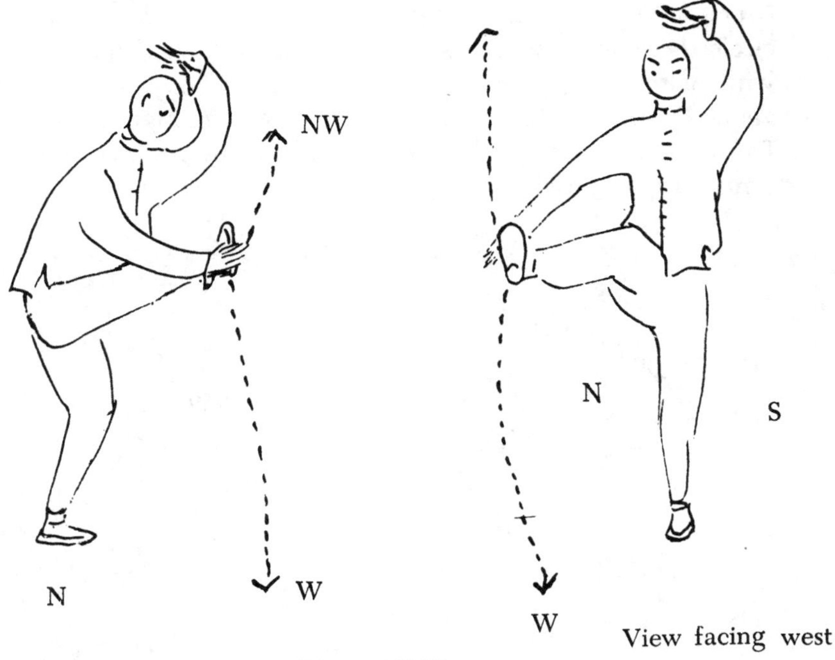

Figure 154B

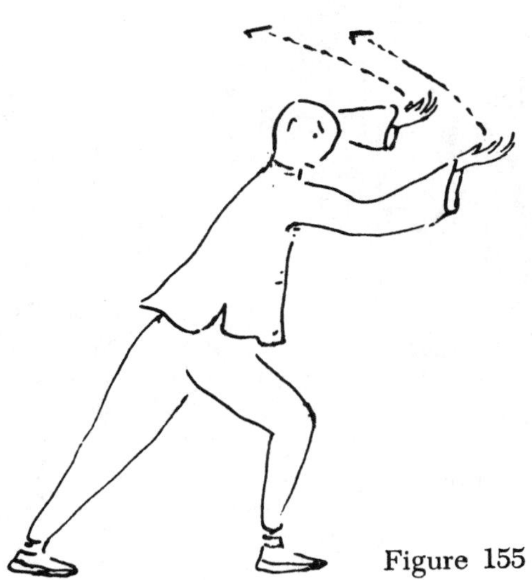

Figure 155

Form 104. Curve Bow Shoot Tiger WAN KUNG SHE HU

Move hands keeping them twelve inches apart: circle both hands with palms leading upward and over toward southeast. Then circle them down southeast, turning palms down. Then circle them, with palms leading, across and in front of body, up to northwest angle. Palms finish facing north with right arm higher than left arm. Do not move legs, head, or body during this circling movement of arms. (Figures 156 and 157)

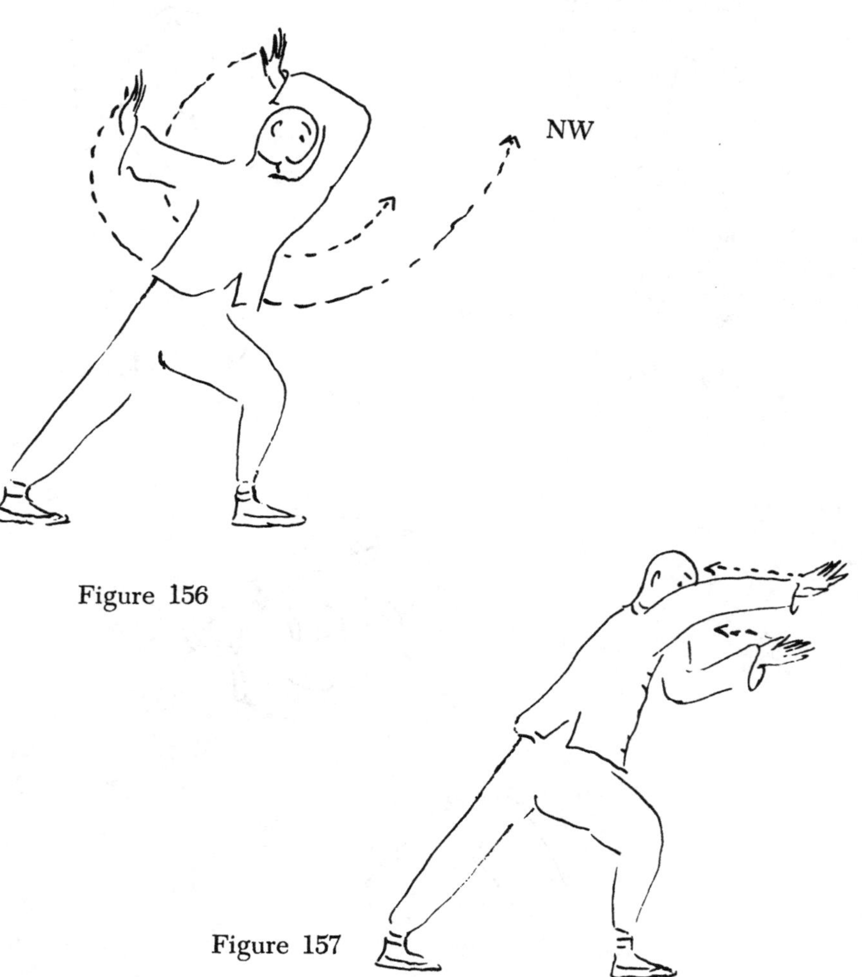

Figure 156

Figure 157

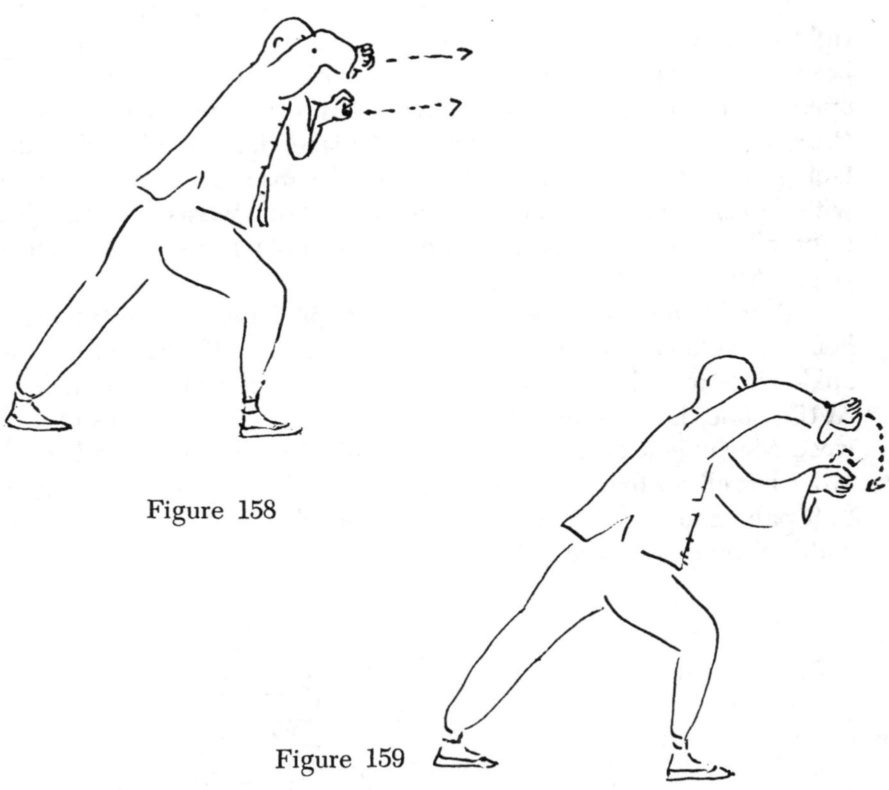

Figure 158

Figure 159

Do not move legs, body, or head. Move both arms at the same time: bend left elbow downward and draw hand, making a fist of it, to left shoulder: fist-palm faces north; wrist is bent so that knuckles of fist are directed west. Bend right elbow, keeping it high, pointing to north, and draw hand, making a fist of it, eye high, to side of face. Wrist is bent so that fist-palm faces north and knuckles point west. (Figure 158)

Do not move legs, head, or body. Move both arms outward to west, each on its own level: right is eye high and left is shoulder high. Fist-palms remain facing north. Fists stop in the same vertical plane, with right arm curved high and left arm angled low. (Figure 159)

Form 105. On Right—High Pat the Horse KAO T'AN MA

Same as Form 34, Figure 68

Shift weight back onto left leg, bending knee and straightening right knee: twist torso to face south; keep right foot on floor; keep head facing west. At the same time both arms move: gradually opening both fists, circle right hand outward and left hand inward. Bring right hand under left arm and place right hand with palm facing down at left armpit. Left arm circles over right, elbow bends with forearm on a diagonal toward floor. Both wrists are straight: right elbow points west and left elbow points east. Head looks west. (Figure 160)

Turn torso to face west and shift weight forward onto right leg, bending its knee, and straighten left knee. Draw left foot with loose ankle close to right foot and place left toes on floor near right foot. At the same time, circle right arm toward west as torso turns to face west. Move right arm high so that hand faces south at head level. Move left elbow to left hip, turning palm up. Both wrists are straight. Left palm and right elbow are on same level; arms are separated by width of body. (Figure 68)

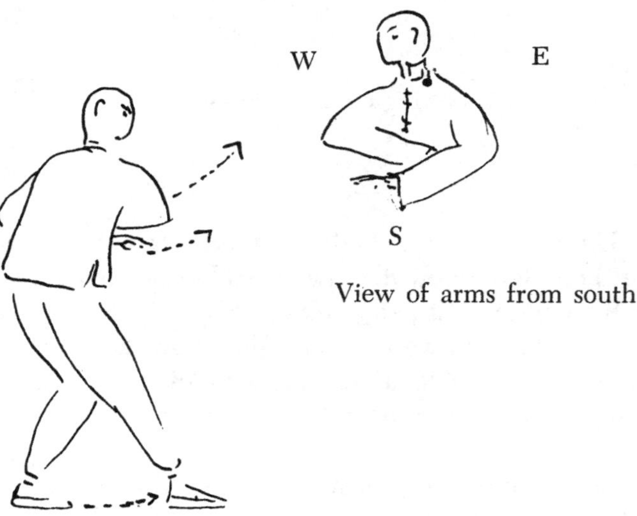

Figure 160

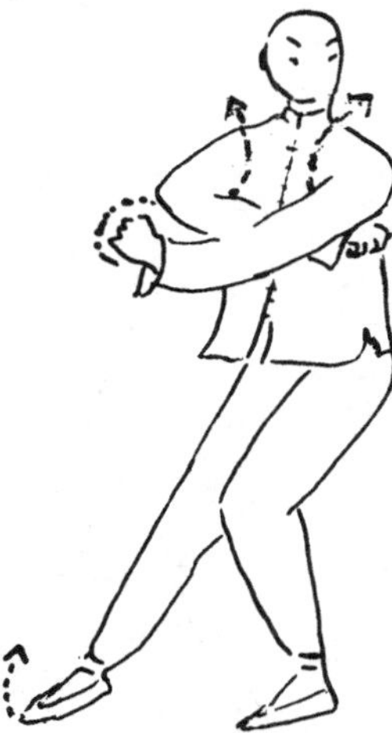

Figure 161

Form 106. Side Face Fist—and Turn Body

P'I MIEN CH'ÜAN CHUAN SHEN

Same as Form 95, Figure 135

Place left heel forward west in the Walking Step Space; transfer weight onto left leg bending knee and straightening right knee. Body is on a slant forward west. At the same time both arms move: place right hand, making it into a fist, at left armpit: fist-palm faces down and elbow is high. Move left arm forward west in line with left shoulder, turn palm to west with fingers pointing up. (Figure 135 with right *fist* instead of open hand)

Keep weight on left leg with its bent knee. Turn left toes inward to point north. Torso turns north and left arm moves with body: gradually straighten wrist and make a fist with fist-palm facing floor. Do not move right arm. (Figure 136)

Move right heel inward, bending right knee slightly. Then move left heel outward to west and straighten right knee. Left arm moves in a horizontal circle with fist approaching right shoulder. (Figure 161)

Quickly move left fist under right arm to right armpit; then in quick sequence remove right fist from left armpit making it go above left shoulder; next in quick succession move left fist in front of left shoulder and right fist in front of right shoulder. These movements—left fist, right fist, and left and right fists—move in succession very speedily. Turn both palms and at the same time slowly open hands to face east; elbows point downward. (Figure 162)

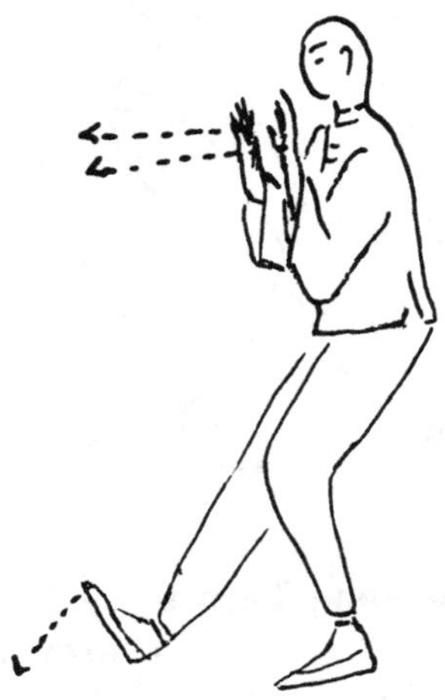

Figure 162

As the quick movements are being done, keep your feet moving in the Toe-Heel-Heel step in the usual basic tempo, turning torso to face east. While both hands are opening slowly, flex right foot, straightening right knee. Weight is on left leg with its bent knee. (Figure 162)

Form 107. Carry Tiger, Push Mountain PAO HU T'UI SHAN

Reverse of Form 14, Figures 33, 34

Shift weight onto right leg forward east, bending right knee and straightening left. At the same time, push both hands, which face east, forward shoulder high to east, each arm in line with its shoulder. Wrists are shoulder high; fingers point upward; body slants forward east. (Figure 33, but in reverse: to east and on right leg)

Keep weight on right leg with its bent knee. Bend torso forward and down, moving arms at the same time. Arms are lowered so that palms face floor at knee level. Arms are perpendicular to floor. (Figure 34, but in reverse: to east and on right leg)

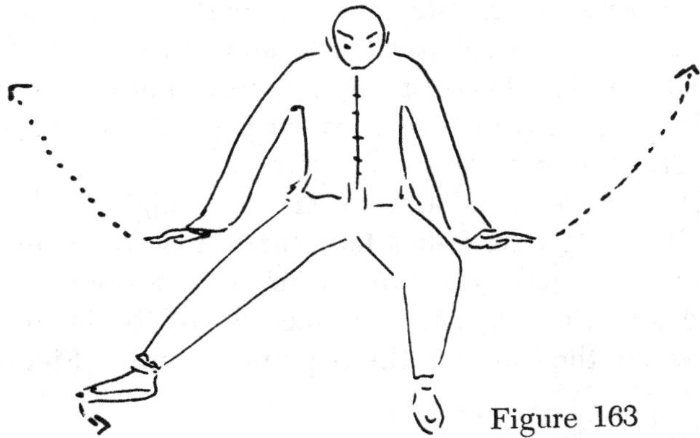

Figure 163

Form 108. Closing Form of T'ai Chi Ch'üan HE T'AI CHI

Turn left toes to north. At the same time shift weight onto left leg bending its knee and straighten right knee. With these movements move torso to north, still remaining bent over. As you move left toes, move left arm to left side of left leg, with palm facing floor and fingers to west. Right hand remains at right side with palm facing floor and fingers to east. (Figure 163)

Turn right toes to north and at the same time, lift torso up to an upright position and with it bring both arms up sideways to shoulder height. As arms move upward, gradually straighten wrists. (Figure 164)

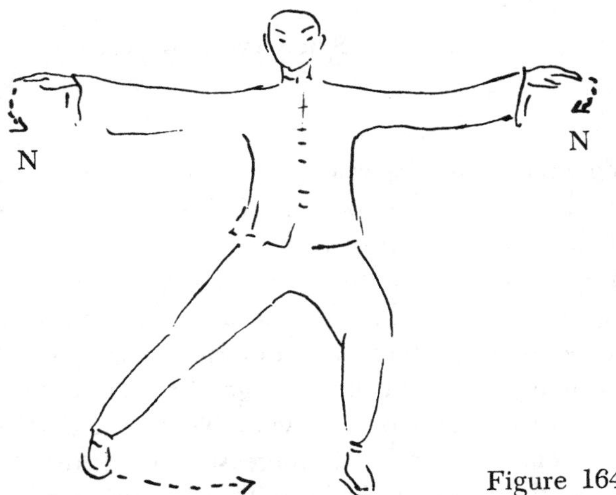

Figure 164

Keep weight on left leg with its bent knee. Move both arms forward at shoulder height to north: hands face floor; wrists are straight; arms are shoulder width apart. At the same time, move right foot and place it parallel to and apart from left foot in your basic stance. Both knees are equally bent. Back is straight.

Keeping arms in their forward parallel position shoulder high, gradually straighten knees. (Figure 165)

Then, lower both arms to sides of thighs, right to right side, and left to left side. Palms face south and wrists are straight. You are now in exactly the same form and position with which you started T'ai Chi Ch'üan. Your feet should be in exactly the same place where they were in the Beginning Form. (Figure 1)

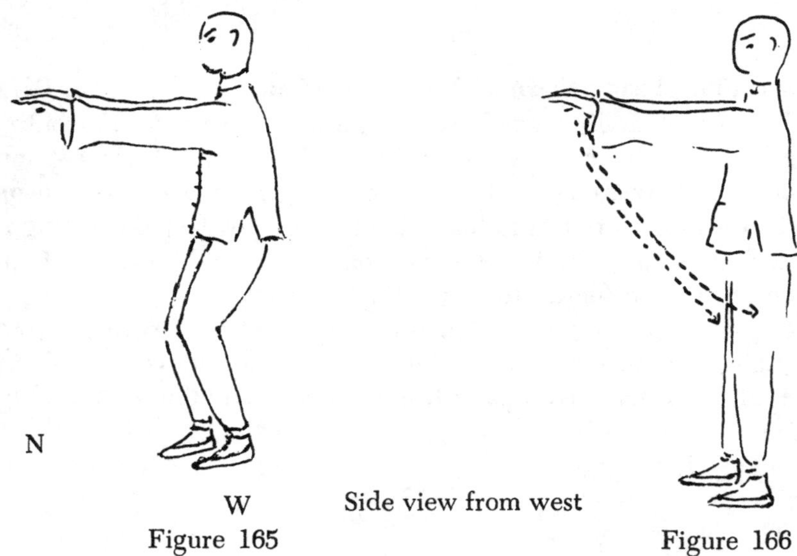

Figure 165

Figure 166

When you finish the entire exercise, remain standing quietly in position, holding the last posture. Release from this position when you "feel" like moving out of it.

This exercise is to be done on the left side, too. When you are proficient and perform the exercise in even tempo, flowingly and continuously, then you may learn it on the reverse side. To study it in this way will augment your knowledge of the subtle details, sharpen your concentration, and perfect your balance and skill. When you perform it relatively well, to increase your interest further you should try to do it very quickly, within ten minutes.

APPENDIX

HISTORICAL BACKGROUND: A CONSISTENT HERITAGE

A great creator of a great work may be considered to represent the culmination of the spirit of his age. In crediting the philosopher Chang San-Feng of the Sung Dynasty (circa eleventh century) with being the father of T'ai Chi Ch'üan, this indeed may be true. Chang San-Feng reflected in his work the intellectual (Confucian) and the spiritual-mystical (Taoist) speculations at that time. He changed and expanded the various exercise systems existing in his day, by creating new forms and techniques, and integrating structure with a style which evolved from his deep experiences and philosophical observances.

The principles that are the very heart of T'ai Chi Ch'üan were derived from the theories and practices of the different ancient Chinese philosophic schools concerned with the development of man's intrinsic and potential powers. Though intriguing subtleties as to man's ultimate destiny may have divided one school from another, all seem to have agreed upon the fact that it was necessary to achieve both heart-calm (tranquillity) and physical health, in order to become a stable, a harmonious, a realized man. Over the centuries since 2000 B.C., philosophers and physicians, alchemists and athletes, have offered their various theories and techniques on: (1) how to combat illnesses of mind and body; (2) how to create the skill to maintain one's health; (3) how to increase one's power and potentialities; (4) and, after restoring the body to its proper harmony, how to open the way to the understanding of qualities hidden deeply in the nature of man—to make him an instrument of his own will.

Even from the earliest times in China, a distinction was made among various forms and functions of designed body-action: (1) those created for commemorative and ritual purposes; (2) those that were intended to stimulate and influence the minds and hearts of the audience; (3) those used to stimulate and direct the feelings, body, and the mind of the doer himself. These last were termed medical or health gymnastic movement. Along with arithmetic, music, writing, and dance for ceremony, the dance for health was included in the liberal arts.

Whatever expressive form the "act of moving" had taken—whether it was the ancient ritual where the priests and shamans danced to honor the "spirits"; or whether, as in communal dance it was to express joy because of a fine harvest—each unmistakably contributed to the idea that body-movement, rhythmically arranged and styled according to physiological and emotional principles, can correct body ills and perpetuate the life force in man.

In ancient China, during Emperor Yü's time (2205 B.C.) stagnant waters from a devastating flood had infested the land. Suspecting that the contamination had resulted from such stagnation, he ordered that a series of exercises, called the Great Dances, be done regularly by all the people. The reasoning was simple and obvious: if inactive waters became diseased, the same could be true of inactive bodies. By doing exercises to stimulate the circulation of the blood, the body would be constantly refreshed, which would make the body impervious to disease. Emperor Yü doubtless was putting into practice theories on circulation inherited from his ancestors who believed that "the blood current flows continuously in a circle and never stops . . . it flows like the current of a river . . . the heart regulates all the blood of the body . . . unceasing circle movement which is life—circulation is the vital current." These are concepts from the year 2600 B.C. (according to the Classic of Medicine, *Nei Ching*, compiled in the third century B.C.) with which our modern world agrees, and are the scientific basis of the physical structure of T'ai Chi Ch'üan.

These ancient dances dictated by Yü thus appear to have evolved from inventions of movement for the cure of diseases a thousand years earlier. Though healing with herbs and plants is known to have been practiced even prior to 3000 B.C., exercise persisted as an essential, necessary part of curative and preventative medicine. Nearly every medical prescription had its related exercise, but there were many more exercises than medical recipes.

That "prevention was the best cure" was known in ancient China and, in a practical sense, may have been the inspiration for the many self-health-exercise systems, since it was said: "Medicine was useful only in *curing* disease."

It was believed that "worry and anxiety cause sickness because they hinder breathing, thus interfering with blood circulation"; so to do exercises for the physical body only was not enough to insure health. "If the mind is peaceful every joint will feel good . . . and joy quickens the circulation" are evidences of the belief that body and mind inextricably affect each other.

Confucius said that the *virtuous* live long. The definition of being virtuous, in this case, included having a peaceful heart, a good body, and an active mind, and with such balanced personality, "one's behaviour could not possibly be improper."

Many streams of philosophic thought contributed to the development of body and mind in harmony, whether it was for "immortality," for long life, or for a better life. All schools included systematic regimes to neutralize the body, by making it so healthy that it would not disturb the mind's growth. "Fatigue your body and you exhaust your mind" was a maxim that clearly compressed this idea of body-mind relationship, as did "clear the intellect and prolong life." The early Taoists (fifth century B.C.), withdrawing from active society, stressed the observation of nature and natural phenomena as an essential part of their philosophy. This interest led them, among other things, to the study of man's movements in relation to the way he functions physically, emotionally, intellectually, and spiritually. Over the many centuries their followers evolved patterns, postures, rhythmic movements and breathing exercises that were intended "to develop a clear intellect, ensure good health, and cure complaints."

Complaints, such as indigestion, asthma, sciatica, tuberculosis, heart ailments, eye and skin diseases (to mention but a few of the "hundred illnesses") could be relieved, so it was claimed, by specialized postures and exercises done systematically. Remedies for mental and emotionl disturbances were given equal consideration. Bad or disquieting dreams, grief, languor, and "ills of the heart," seemingly baseless fears, indolence, "liking savoury things," and insanity were carefully prescribed for. Man's mental, physical, and emotional health were always considered together, as an entity.

In the early centuries B.C., of immense importance were the techniques to develop the skill in maintaining health and the power to improve it. Gymnastic exercise, or medical movement, besides being a remedy for disease, was made a branch of education for the healthy person as well. "As a means to long life," said Chuang Tzu (fourth century B.C.), philosopher of the Taoist school, "pass some time like a dormant bear." "Imitate the flappings of a duck, the ape's dance, the owl's fixed stare, the tiger's crouch, the pawings of a bear," said others in this time (from a Taoist notebook by Edward Herbert). There was no school of thought, alchemy, medicine, which did not include physical culture as a basic necessity for health and spirituality.

The term applied to medical exercises is *Kung-Fu,* meaning "work-man" or "work-done," implying that the man himself does the remedial work for himself. It is not imposed upon him from the outside by doctors or masseurs; this was considered by some to be a "degraded form of body training." The conscious control which he exerts upon himself is the most advantageous method for "self-improvement." It was believed that "the mechanism is assisted by placing the body in many different attitudes and postures, in assorted positions of all kinds," and that such combinations produce healthful physiological changes, these to be used to treat diseases; and that, by isolation and nonmovement of one part in relation to another moving part, profound improvements would result.

The study of what movements to combine, what to separate, what particular articulations are necessary, resulted in an enormous number of arrangements, permutations, and combinations. To these were added a system of breathing and various positions of lying, standing, sitting, moving (leaps, runs, walks, etc.), combining the elements of activity and passivity. Kung-Fu accomplishes the cure of infirmities, restores harmony in the body, and therefore man, when not disturbed by irregularities, "is freed from the servitude of the senses." The roots of T'ai Chi Ch'üan are embedded in the rich soil of such thought.

In the third century of this era, Hua T'o, a surgeon who had experimented with anesthetics, stressed the physical and emotional values of exercise. In a lecture to one of his disciples (as recorded in the *History of Chinese Medicine* by Drs. K. C. Wong and Wu Lien-Teh), Hua T'o said, "The body needs exercise, only it must not be done to the point of exhaustion.... It promotes free circulation of the blood and prevents sickness. The used doorstep never rots, so the body. That is why the ancients practiced the bear's neck ... and moving the joints to prevent old age. I have a system of exercise called the frolics of the five animals ... the tiger, deer, bear, monkey, and bird. It removes disease, strengthens the legs, and ensures health. If one *feels out of sorts,* just practice one of these frolics. ..." "To promote sweating and to give feeling of lightness," jumping, twisting, swaying, crawling, swinging contractions and extensions were prescribed, and it was recommended that they be done regularly. Later systems, as was T'ai Chi Ch'üan, were guided by the principle that the exercise which is truly health-promoting must never exhaust or fatigue, but, on the contrary, should build up a greater energy and should produce a feeling of contentment.

Between the second and the tenth centuries A.D., innumerable gymnastic systems evolved, each specially created for specific purposes. Especially important were the technical contributions made by the many "religious" sects, each in its own secret society. Inasmuch as there had been no medical or philosophical systems that did not include physical culture, these sects, too, made the training of the body an indispensable requirement, for becoming a sage and for health and longevity. In the philosophy of Lao-Tzu (sixth century B.C.) are admonitions for using one's superior abilities for the common good of society. Different secret groups, at various periods in China's long history, put their physical skills to practical use, "to improve the world and better the lives of the people." An instance of this is the activity of the Yellow Turbans, a sect that aided the final fall of the decaying Han Dynasty at the end of the second century A.D. They fought unarmed, because no "common people" were allowed to carry weapons at this time. Fighting in "unarmed combat" required special techniques and rigorous training, which necessitated the development of new forms and styles. What is important to stress as being pertinent to T'ai Chi Ch'üan is the fact with these physical disciplines, the principle that mind and body together produce perfect prowess was never forgotten.

Inevitably, by the fourth century, with a background of a thousand years of intensive consideration given to physical-mental health, many separate styles matured, each proclaiming its own physiological and philosophical point of view. A fourth-century boxer wrote a "Canon for Developing the Sinews." Another wrote a treatise on "Deep Breathing As It Relates to Movement." "Lessons for Tensing Movements" became very popular. Exercises in slow and fast tempi were experimented with. Posture-attitudes, allied to philosophy, became an important part of various cults. All were designed for the improvement of health, physical, mental, and spiritual.

None of these forms was ever associated with the arts, because the different objectives of dance and gymnastic were never lost sight of or confused. Nevertheless these exercises had a structural form and a designed composition which we have come to associate with art, and which contribute vitally to the final objective of experiencing an emotional satisfaction and a sense of equilibrium.

In the sixth century, when Buddhist influences, merging with Taoist thought, impregnated the art of painting and the philosophy of ideas and behavior, an Indian monk (called Ta Mo in China) settled down in China at the Shao Lin Monastery. It appears that at this particular period, in contrast to the preceding centuries, and in this particular retreat, the monks were not aware of the necessity of having physical health in order to attain mystical experience. Ta Mo instituted a series of systematic exercises to revivify the enfeebled and emaciated monks, mentally and physically. His Eighteen Form Lohan Exercise, he said, "would transform the body into a strong abode, to provide the soul with a dwelling place." Named for the monastery, his Shao Lin style represents the technique of the "outer-extrinsic" school of exercise (*Wai Chia*). In this "outer" type, muscular action is intense and visible, dynamics are strong and unvaried, energy is external and forcibly produced. Although primarily used for self-defense purposes and for wrestling, it is also practiced today as a personal exercise, since this style too includes the aim of becoming tranquil, as well as being strong.

Another point of view as to what "way of movement" could best prolong life and rejuvenate it was being formulated at this time. Called the soft "inner-intrinsic" school (*Nei Chia*), this technique gave rise to various styles that are in practice today.

It is known that during the T'ang Dynasty (circa A.D. 750) several different kinds of Kung-Fu (not yet called Ch'üan) were in practice. A long-bearded philosopher, Hsü Hsuan-P'ing (a wood cutter by trade) performed a "Long Kung-Fu," in which the patterns were continuously connected. The ingredients of *length* and *continuity* added a new element to the philosophy of mental discipline and to the science of increasing physical endurance. Of the thirty-seven Forms comprising his Long Kung-Fu, Hand Strums the Lute, Single Whip, Seven Stars, Jade Girl, High-Pat the Horse, Phoenix (Stork or Crane in today's version) Flaps Its Wings, are Forms that are in T'ai Chi Ch'üan today. During this period several other Kung-Fu having this character of "continuity" were being practiced: "Heavenly-Inborn," "Nine Small Heavens" and "Acquired Kung-Fu." These early forms were the seeds from which the 108 Forms of T'ai Chi Ch'üan flowered.

By the Sung Dynasty (after A.D. 1000), the concept of "the inner-intrinsic" school (*Nei Chia*) was firmly established. This system emphasized "soft" movement as being the best technique for loosening the joints, circulating the blood, and building up a reserve of energy, with the philosophy that the mind must be in control of action, and that through this method, since "man was capable of wonders," he could fulfill himself as a superior, a "realized" human being. Of the many philosophers engaged in the pursuit of such fulfillment, and who consistently practiced various Ch'üan, was Chang San-Feng, who was over ninety when he died.

He was sixty-seven years old, when, after thirty-five years of study, he settled down at the Wu Tang Monastery for nine years. During this time he created his version of Ch'üan, and his "way" was completed. Linking older Forms, changing and augmenting them, he evolved a unified system utilizing the principle of the T'ai Chi, which, when in action, separates into Yin and Yang. They say that he was inspired by the play of the contrasting movements of the bird and the serpent—the firm and the yielding. Alternating Yin and Yang in continuous succession, and with the principle of "controlling the active by means of the quiet," he created his Ch'üan from the point of view of philosophy and physiology, psychology, geometry and the law of dynamics. Opposed to hardness, he stressed elasticity, and made a distinction between nature giving strength (physical) and man giving strength (will-power).

His inner-intrinsic school of exercise (*Nei Chia*) is known as the Wu Tang school from the monastery where it was, so to speak, synthesized. This vital system is said to embrace the most permanent, profound, and scientific aspects of its predecessors. Its scope was extended to include a technique for heightening perception and increasing the ability to concentrate and co-ordinate, of activating the mind, and of producing a harmonious equilibrium of thought and action for the attainment of tranquillity. The concept of *T'ai Chi Ch'üan* dates from Chang San-Feng's time.

The various styles (see page 4) came into being during the ensuing centuries. The Wu Style is a variation of the original Yang Style and was created by Wu Yü. The other styles also take their names from their originators. Mr. Ma Yüeh-Liang (my teacher of the Wu style) believes that "some creations are improvements of previous inventions and are better than the former because the new ones have been able to eliminate mistakes and have had more time to perfect themselves."

Chang San-Feng's theories were documented and augmented by Wang Chung-Yüeh (Ming Dynasty, circa fifteenth century). Following are excerpts from his book and two other documents attributed to this period. (These were translated for me by Koo Hsien-Liang, Hubert Wang, and Sally Ch'eng.)

EXCERPTS FROM MING DYNASTY DOCUMENTS

1. *T'ai Chi Ch'üan Ching* (Classic) by Wang Chung-Yüeh.

T'ai Chi is infinity, the absolute; it creates from "no limit." It contains dynamic and static movement; it is the mother of Yin and Yang, of everything male and female. It is the root of motion, which is division, and of stillness, which is union. It must neither be overdone nor underdone—it must be exact. . . . Comprehension comes from growing understanding plus effort and this leads one gradually to full enlightenment. Unless one pursues this exercise long enough one cannot hope to understand fully. . . .

Be open-minded (receptive-void) and concentrate on the top of the head, with Ch'i marshaled in the abdomen. Lean in either direction and be "as if suddenly hiding, suddenly appearing." If left side is weighted it is then ready to change to void (Hsü); if right side is weighted (Shih), then it is ready to change to void. . . . When one looks from below upward at a T'ai Chi Ch'üan master, he appears to be lofty. The longer you look, the loftier he appears. When you look at him from above downward, he looks more "deep." . . . A feather cannot be added, nor a fly land without effecting a change (in balance). . . . When a master stands he is in perfect balance and moves as a carriage wheel does. . . . If one doesn't progress, it is probably one's own fault because of bad habits. . . . One must know Yin and Yang; Yin does not leave Yang and Yang does not leave Yin; they mutually help each other. . . . Thus it is that comprehension (understanding plus effort) leads to skill. By quietly studying and analyzing, one gradually learns to do—at the bidding of the mind. Theoretically one should forget oneself and learn from others. The prevailing mistake is to seek things which one is not yet equipped to learn. By making even a tiny mistake, one can go wrong a thousand miles. This leads dangerously to endless blunders. Beginners would do well to bear this in mind and should study discriminatingly.

2. *Shih-San Shih Ko:* Song of the Thirteen Kinetic Movements (ward off slantingly upward, pushing, pressing forward or squeezing, pushing downward, gathering, twisting, elbowing, leaning, stepping forward, stepping backward, looking right, looking left, and being centered). Never neglect any of the thirteen kinetic changes.

All important thought should be aimed at the vital junctures. You must be attentive to the slightest change from Hsü (empty) to Shih (solid). . . . A movement has its seeds in the state of stillness before it is seen. . . . In every movement one must analyze the hidden meaning. When well-done all appears effortless. Pay attention to the waist at all times. With abdomen loose and light, Ch'i can move (be in full swing). If coccyx is properly centered, the "spirit" rises from the top of the head. Body is so light that only head matters. If you pay attention to the push and pull, expansion-contraction, bend and stretch, open and close, you will then have full freedom and you can do anything you like. (Beginners best be guided by oral teaching.) Work incessantly and skill will take care of itself. What is meant by making good use of the body? The answer is the mind wills and the body obeys (guiding spirit-mind is the master and the body—bones and flesh—is the servant). Think what the final purpose is—that one will never grow old (spring will be eternal).... If you do not search in this direction, it will be a sheer waste of effort and that would be such a pity!

3. *Shih-San Shih Hsing-Kung Hsin Chieh:* Treatise on the Thirteen Kinetic Movements As They Relate to Mental Comprehension.

Calmness is of decisive importance... there will be perfect spontaneity only when everything is done according to the dictates of the mind. There will be no danger of being heavy and clumsy, or of not attaining lightness (at top of head) if the spirit co-operates.

Facility of action comes from change of movements from Hsü to Shih (from void to solid). Even when exerting effort one must be calm and appear effortless. One must concentrate and aim at one direction. The entire body must be loose, straight, comfortable, peaceful, quiet, centered.... One must be prepared to face any change in the eight directions.... Motion should be like refined steel. The form is like that of a hawk about to seize a rabbit; the spirit is like that of a cat about to catch a mouse. The quietness is like that of a mountain range; movement is agile, like a river.

Storing up energy is like that of an open bow; letting go (of effort-energy) is like that of letting the arrow go. Seek straightness in a curve. Store up energy before using it. Strength comes from the spine; steps follow body changes. Getting ready is as important as doing. It has continuity, though it has "broken movement." Like a pleat which folds in on itself and continues to the next one with rhythm and order, so the movement goes forward and back with rhythm and order and continuity. There must be changes, alterations, and variety. Only when one knows how to be "soft" can one be properly strong. Learn to breathe well and then you will have alacrity-alertness-speed. Ch'i must be cultivated without hindrance, as a result of which you will be able to do anything. Stamina is stored up, is saved, by moving in curves. The mind gives the orders (is in command); the breath is the banner; the waist is the leader (the hinge, the axis).

First learn to stretch and expand; then learn to contract and condense.... Then it will be possible to be perfectly integrated (be a master).

First conceive in the mind; then express in the body. Keep abdomen loose; breath permeates bones; give spirit free rein and the body will be calm. Be attentive all the time. Deeply remember: one single movement suffices to effect the whole body movement; there is no isolated quiet without enveloping the whole being.... Inside, one is firm, and outside, one shows peacefulness. The even pace is like that of a cat walking. The strength exerted is like that of pulling silk. One's attention is on the spirit, not on the breath... too much preoccupation with breath makes one clumsy. ... The appearance of "lack of breath" is real strength....

Authors of special books on T'ai Chi Ch'üan (to whom I referred, as translated for me by Hubert Wang and Koo Hsien-Liang) are: Wu Chien Ch'üan and Ma Yüeh-Liang, Tung Ying-Chieh, Ts'ai Ho Peng (a compilation), Wu T'u Nan, Ch'ang Ch'un, Hsü Chih-Yi, Dr. Ch'ü Mien-Yü.